POEMS FROM THE MEDICAL WORLD

Poems from the Medical World

A Falcon House Anthology

Edited by

Howard Sergeant

MTP PRESS LIMITED
International Medical Publishers

Published by

MTP Press Limited
Falcon House
Lancaster, England

British Library Cataloguing in Publication Data

Poems from the medical world.
1. Medicine – Poetry 2. English poetry
I. Sergeant, Howard
821'.008'031 PR1195.M/

ISBN 0-85200-289-0

Printed and bound by
REDWOOD BURN LIMITED
Trowbridge and Esher

Phototypesetting by Rainbow Graphics, Liverpool

Contents

Acknowledgements

Acknowledgements are due to the poets who have allowed their work to be reprinted or included here, and to the following publications and anthologies in which some of the poems first appeared:

Allusions (University of Lancaster), *Anglo-Welsh Review, Encounter, Envoi, Lancet, Ludd's Mill, Meridian, New Poetry, Nursing Mirror, Outposts, Other Poetry, Parents Voice, Pick,* and *Poetry and Audience* and *New Poems 1977/78, New Poetry 4, Poems 1975 Ver Poets,* and Surrey Poetry Centre.

For permission to reproduce poems the Editor and Publishers are indebted to the following:

Agenda Editions for the four poems from *Mortal Fire* by Peter Dale.

Cape Golliard for "Learning to Breathe" and "An Accident" from *Trampoline* by Gael Turnbull.

Hutchinson & Co Ltd., for "The Smile Was", "Pathology of Colours", and "The Stethoscope" from *Collected Poems* by Dannie Abse.

Keepsake Press for "Old Age of a Clown" and "Faster than Light" from *Poetry and Paradox* by Edward Lowbury.

Manifold Chapbooks for "Old Man in a Home" and "On a Death in an Old People's Home" from *Midway This Path* by May Ivimy.

Mitre Press for "Blood Transfusion" and "Post-Mortem" from *Snow Children* by S. L. Henderson Smith.

Outposts Publications for "The Village Doctor" and "The Library" from *Give me the Hill-Run Boys* by Margaret Gillies; for "Emergency Room" from *Intimations* and "The Operation" from *Glimmerings* by S. L. Henderson Smith; and for all the poems by Henry Shore from *Selected Poems*.

Peterloo Poets for "The Visitors" and "Farewell, Gibson Square" from *A Lifetime of Dying* by Elizabeth Bartlett, and "Job Description" and "For Saint Peter" from *Side Effects* by U. A. Fanthorpe.

The Executors of the Estate of Lord Russell Brain for all the poems included here from *Poems and Verses* (privately printed).

'Man is the Shuttle'

Man

Weighing the steadfastness and state
Of some mean things which here below reside,
Where birds like watchful clocks the noiseless date
And intercourse of times divide,
Where bees at night get home and hive, and flowers
Early, as well as late,
Rise with the sun, and set in the same bowers;

I would (said I) my God would give
The staidness of these things to man! for these
To his divine appointments ever cleave,
And no new business breaks their peace;
The birds nor sow, nor reap, yet sup and dine,
The flowers without clothes live,
Yet Solomon was never dressed so fine.

Man hath still either toys, or care,
He hath no root, nor to one place is tied,
But ever restless and irregular
About this earth doth run and ride,
He knows he hath a home, but scarce knows where,
He says it is so far
That he hath quite forgot how to go there.

He knocks at all doors, strays and roams,
Nay, hath not so much wit as some stones have,
Which in the darkest nights point to their homes
By some hid sense their Maker gave;
Man is the shuttle, to whose winding quest
And passage through these looms
God ordered motion, but ordained no rest.

HENRY VAUGHAN

Drinking

The thirsty earth soaks up the rain,
And drinks and gapes for drink again;
The plants suck in the earth, and are
With constant drinking fresh and fair;
The sea itself (which one would think
Should have but little need of drink)
Drinks ten thousand rivers up,
So filled that they o'erflow the cup.
The busy Sun (and one would guess
By's drunken fiery face no less)
Drinks up the sea, and when he's done,
The Moon and Stars drink up the Sun:
They drink and dance by their own light,
They drink and revel all the night:
Nothing in Nature's sober found,
But an eternal health goes round.
Fill up the bowl, then, fill it high,
Fill all the glasses there—for why
Should every creature drink but I?
Why, man of morals, tell me why?

ABRAHAM COWLEY

Urban Pollution

Ye who amid this feverish world would wear
A body free of pain, of cares a mind;
Fly the rank city, shun its turbid air;
Breathe not the chaos of eternal smoke
And volatile corruption, from the dead,
The dying, sickening, and the living world
Exhaled, to sully Heaven's transparent dome
With dim mortality. It is not air
That from a thousand lungs reeks back to thine,
Sated with exhalations rank and fell,
The spoil of dunghills, and the putrid thaw
Of nature; when from shape and texture she
Relapses into fighting elements:
It is not air, but floats a nauseous mass
Of all obscene, corrupt, offensive things.

JOHN ARMSTRONG

A Cloud of Ghosts

This city is haunted by young men without ambition,
Who don't seem to care about girls, or motor-cars,
Or holding any sort of position.
    There is a timeless air about them:
Whether in hotel bars,
Knocking back Scotch with a serious air,
Saying the world is as well without them;
Or, in the afternoon, at coffee,
Earthing dreams we would not dare,
For fear of shock, attempt,
They stir round their mysterious coffee
The giant current of the soul,
And hold themselves in all exempt,
Rather than one should say aloof,
From common things. Yet they pay toll,
If not in quantity of time, to weight;
As though each leaden hour must own its proof,
—Futility, or action, or learning—
And leave that marker on the sea of fate,
Filed for future reference.
    Theirs is nameless yearning.
A pause in search of commas
To end the awful inference
Of silence. A shy dream,
Summoning some long-forgotten promise
To be true. Only this,
Grafted across a moonbeam
In a deserted street
In the metropolis,
Or hung across the evening sun
Before it can retreat
Through the West End park;
And the fat dragon of the lonely one
That will slide away
Into the sliding dark,
And leave the weary plaintiff there to mourn.

Yesterday,
A hint of paradise in nameless places;
Or glimpsing peace in some sequestered bourne;
While tomorrow
Eats into the same faces
With the same mixture of sullen joy
And treasured sorrow.
It is surely many times that they have vowed,
I will be my father's son. I will employ
Reason. I will accept the surfaces
I'm told I touch, and be a doctor. Do him proud.
Wipe the skies clean and study God;
Or, without any dilatory prefaces,
Build my business like a man, and charge far
Into eternity—And then they'll nod,
And smile wisely on each other—
Here's enough to tip the verger,
They'll say. You won't make more than that.
Where were we before you interrupted, brother?
—Eh?
What were we looking at?
So, by suffering a flame
To burn enamel off clay,
They prise the core of things apart,
And find a same
Substantive, a same gasp
That the most inner heart
In the electric storm of birth
Must importunely clasp,
And with bright forms and phantom shapes
People earth.
They never know enough.
They keep on making passes through the drapes,
Till one day, drawing blood,
They find a different stuff,
Reached at the very point of all their wonder.
Then they may daub their dribbling wounds with mud,
And seal the flame in place with broken ice,
And stamp the mist of memory with thunder.

Over those unrepenting ranks
No banner flies, and no device
Tells what they would do.
No one comes to offer thanks
For helping out humanity
When life's worn through.
I am haunted by a vision of their lonely urge to truth,
Their total disregard for human vanity.
Why is it all the things we spend a lifetime doing
Seem all at once unlovely, and uncouth?
—We live in hope that we do greater things
Than we shall ever know. Old time is brewing
Our black draught of death. How summers go!
How seventy we are before it springs!
. . . And a haven hard to come by.
They are the unsung overflow
Who void our gambling proposition,
Denounce the deadline 'Live, or die!',
And the exclamation-marks of rain
In the painted clouds of false ambition.
Through the vacuum where they go,
Where they can never go again,
A ghost cloud shivers in the empty air,
Just like a rainbow on the snow,
Staining our eyes with stuff that isn't there.

RUSSELL GRANT

An Accident

As I ran to catch a bus, my heart fell out. This was
quite painless, but I was startled as you might
imagine.

It didn't appear to have been damaged. Feeling rather
sheepish, I picked it up and put it in my pocket.

No one seemed to have noticed but when I got on to
the next bus some school children at the back
began to giggle.

How could they tell? Is this a common occurrence?
Should I call a doctor?

Meanwhile, I keep it in the refrigerator. This is
a warm summer. If it should spoil, I might
have trouble getting another.

GAEL TURNBULL

A Great Talker

(for Ron Page)

Ron talked continuously
to a complete stranger
for over an hour and a half
on every subject under the sun:
football teams, family ties,
photography, philanthropy,
the weather predictably enough,
prices of every kind of stuff
he could think of, cars,
beers in bottles or cans.
He plied him with Player's
filtertip fags when I knew
he had only a few left.
Ron even had the audacity
to ask him who he voted
for at the general election.
Normally I would have asked him
to shut up but who else
would have taken his place
while firemen fought to release
the Guy's trapped leg
from the twisted wreckage.

WILLIAM LINDSAY

Doctors, Clinics and Surgeries

The Village Doctor

He tended his flock
After his own fashion,
Unorthodox at times,
Lancet might not have understood
His language
But we,
The people of the village
Knew just what he meant,
Talking to us with robust and country vigour
Telling the men among us
Many a ribald tale,
Speaking of sport
Rather than ailments.

Children went to him
Like bees to certain honey,
Sometimes feigning illness
When they thought him to be near;
He knew our fears and foibles,
Our problems,
Cured us when he could,
Jollied us through jungles of despair,
Laughed with us, cried with us,
He loved us
Though he never would have said so,
Pooh-poohed all praise
And turned away from it.

Old folk were never left
To feel alone,
Getting unscheduled visits
To cheer their winter's day,
Made sure they needed nothing.
Road accidents he hated
Till it showed,
Once
Rocked in his strong arms
The mutilated body of a child,
Till help came
Crooning
As tenderly as any Mother
Poor wee lamb,
My poor wee lamb.

Felt with a sixth sense
For the feelings
Of a woman in childbirth
And her emerging babe;
Showed unexpected gentleness,
Sighed with satisfaction
At the new cot cuddled bairn
Stating all best babies
Born at home.

Life never lost for him its fascination
Nor he his deep compassion.

MARGARET GILLIES

Portrait of a Physician

Long has he been of that amphibious fry,
Bold to prescribe, and busy to apply.
His shop the gazing vulgar's eyes employs
With foreign trinkets, and domestic toys.
Here, mummies lay most reverendly stale,
And there, the tortoise hung her coat of mail;
Not far from some huge shark's devouring head,
The flying fish their finny pinions spread.
Aloft in rows large poppy heads were strung,
And near, a scaly alligator hung.
In this place, drugs in musty heaps decayed,
In that, dried bladders, and drawn teeth were laid.
An inner room receives the numerous shoals
Of such as pay to be reputed fools.
Globes stand by globes, volumes on volumes lie,
And planitary schemes amuse the eye.

The sage, in velvet chair, here lolls at ease,
To promise future health for present fees.
Then, as from tripod, solemn shams reveals,
And what the stars know nothing of, foretells.
One asks how soon Panthea may be won,
And longs to feel the Marriage fetters on.
Others, convinced by melancholy proof,
Would know how soon kind Fates will strike 'em off.
Some, by what means they may redress the wrong,
When fathers the possession keep too long.
And some would know the issue of their Cause,
And whether gold can sodder up its flaws.
Poor pregnant Laijs his advice would have,
To lose by Art what fruitful Nature gave;
And Portia old in expectation grown,
Laments her barren Curse, and begs a son.

Whilst Iris, his cosmetic wash must try,
To make her bloom revive, and lovers dye.
Some ask for charms, and others philtres choose
To gain Corinna, and their quartans lose.
Young Hylas, botched with stains too foul to name,
In cradle here, renews his youthful frame:
Cloyed with desire, and surfeited with charms,
A hot-house he prefers to Julia's arms.
And old Lucullus would the Arcanum prove,
Of kindling in cold veins the sparks of Love.

SIR SAMUEL GARTH

The Doctor

Guilty, he does not always like his patients.
But here, black fur raised, their yellow-eyed dog
mimics Cerberus, barks barks at the invisible,
so this man's politics, how he may crawl
to superiors does not matter. A doctor must care
and the wife's on her knees in useless prayer,
the young daughter's like a waterfall.

Quiet, Cerberus! Soon enough you'll have a bone
or two. Now, coughing, the patient expects
the unjudged lie: 'Your symptoms are familiar
and benign'—someone to be cheerfully sure,
to transform tremblings, gigantic unease,
by naming like a pet some small disease
with a known aetiology, certain cure.

So the doctor will and yes he will prescribe
the usual dew from a banana leaf; poppies and
honey too; ten snowflakes or something whiter
from the bole of a tree; the clearest water
ever, melting ice from a mountain lake;
sunlight from waterfall's edge, rainbow smoke;
tears from eyelashes of the daughter.

DANNIE ABSE

Farewell, Gibson Square

(for Dr Susan Heath)

We did surgeries together. I warned her
Who liked litigation, and who were devious,
And who were mildly insane.
We managed to break a patient's arm
Between us, when he fell unconscious
To the floor. In the surgery,
I ask you, what shame. True the patient
Was deaf, and didn't hear our questions.
Compassion ended in gusts of laughter.
Not seemly. She wasn't a seemly girl.
Newly qualified, tat became her;
She wasn't sure if medicine
Was her thing. Lying in bed, smoking
And reading, was. She taught me
How to pour a Guinness slowly;
She was pale and slow-spoken, witty
And thin.
Hospitals got her down, she said,
After a while that is,
And furnished rooms made her puke,
But pubs and jumble sales
Were her natural habitat.
At last I heard she'd got a job
In a chest clinic, smoking illicitly
In the toilets, no doubt.
Fair Susan, with your Afro hair style,
Your pot-plants, and your miniscule
Bank balance, I miss you.
Professional boredom has settled in
Again, and patients go home whole.

ELIZABETH BARTLETT

Town Clinics

Herded in clinic cattle-cubicles,
We wait with patience our appointed time;
Unknown to each other
We stay sealed in cocoons of silence;
Neat nurses pass smartly back and forth
On 'squeeching' floors,
Pleasant but with faces
Lacking the light of recognition.
Nothing to do but thumb through old magazines
And watch our fellows;
See the despondency of some, the hope of others;
The anxious Mother pestered by her peevish child
Until in clear tones
Each in turn our names are called
And we disappear behind big, blank,
Close shut doors that break the monotony
Of the long white sterile wall.

Doctors greet us
With long practised voices of confidence
And look out from kind but no contact eyes,
Flick through our files,
Question us a little,
Do what they can to heal the body
But have little time to ease the troubled mind.
It's not their fault,
They, like us, are slaves to the system,
We are file people,
They have their schedules to keep,
Their numbers to get through,
Forms to fill out.

Oh how much rather would I be where I am known
Back in the warm waiting room of the village Doctor
Where I can feel that I am me
And know that I exist.

MARGARET GILLIES

From The Dispensary

As bold Mirmillo the grey dawn descries,
Armed cap-à-pie, where honour calls, he flies,
And finds the legions planted at their post;
Where mighty Querpo fillęd the eye the most.
His arms were made, if we may credit fame,
By Mulciber, the mayor of Birmingham.
Of tempered stibium the bright shield was cast,
And yet the work the metal far surpassed.
A foliage of the vulnerary leaves,
Graved round the brim, the wondering sight deceives.
Around the centre Fate's bright trophies lay,
Probes, saws, incision-knives, and tools to slay.
Embossed upon the field, a battle stood
Of leeches spouting haemorrhoidal blood.
The artist too expressed the solemn state
Of grave physicians at a consult met;
About each symptom how they disagree,
But how unanimous in case of fee.
Whilst each assassin his learned colleague tires
With learned impertinence, the sick expires.
Beneath this blazing orb bright Querpo shone,
Himself an Atlas, and his shield a moon.
A pestle for his truncheon led the van,
And his high helmet was a close-stool pan.

SIR SAMUEL GARTH

Extracts from a Police Surgeon's Notebook

1.
History: arrested for drunken driving
and was carried into the charge room.
Examination: in the Rhomberg test
he complained that the room was going
round and round, almost falling.
Speech incoherent, could not spell his name.
Placed sixteen coins of every kind
in circulation on the table and asked
him to count them as normal procedure
and like lightning, faster than I could,
answered, "8/4½d". Accurate. Occupation:-
barrow-boy.

2.
Unconscious drunk examined re possible injury
but on arrival had made sufficient recovery
to sit up; could not stand without assistance.
Had vomited. Nothing abnormal discovered
other than acute alcoholism. Vigorously denied
being drunk and offered to demonstrate
something that none present could do.
He did. Stood on his head, absolutely upright
for two minutes, arms outright, unwavering.
Occupation claimed:- "Head-case; obvious isn't it".

3.
History: free-wheeling in an old banger
without engine running, started on an incline
at 7 a.m. on a Sunday morning.
Worked all night on a newspaper
where each worker was required to provide
either a bottle of spirits or crate of beer.
Worst driver condition I have seen
as a police surgeon for ten years.
Paralytic. Apologetic. Pleaded guilty
at court at the first hearing
but subsequent analysis of urine
revealed no alcohol in the blood,
a result which leaves me completely mystified.

4.
Driving under influence. Alcotest positive.
"On my life, I'm sober.
Had nothing to drink since last night
when I had a pint.
I've heard you can give blood
from the big toe. Is that so?
All right. Don't get the needle.
I can't stand the sight of blood.
I can't stand when I see a needle.
I faint when I see a needle.
I can't pee in public,
will you look the other way;
the way you look at my pubic
makes you look the *other* way.
My cup is full and running over!
My terylene/worsted are all wet,
I tell you I'm quite sober.
How much fine do you think I'll get?"

WILLIAM LINDSAY

Mother

Margaret had a very low I.Q. but she was a wonderful mother.
Common sense seethed from every pore
And her dense but lovely children clustered 'round my legs
When I opened their front door.

I looked at them, every one destined to be a labourer—
No girls—six boys with sun-blonde hair.
From Tim at eight to Michael at two, in cascading sizes,
They ushered me into a worn, chintz chair.

They showed me this, they showed me that, including Bert (the hamster).
I smiled and said, "He's very nice."
"Of course he is," they cried because he was part of the family
As were the cats and dogs and mice.

I saw young Alan, barely three, with impetigo on his knee
And wrote a script upon my pad.
I gazed at the children standing in a row, amazingly all alike,
And every one had a different dad.

WILLIAM DUNCAN

Miracle Cure

He stumbled from the night
of drums and cicadas
into the lamplit gloom
of a doctor's waiting room . . .
a Bantu boy of twelve,
groping, bumping into chairs.
'What's wrong?' I said. 'My eyes,'
he panted; 'a snake
spat poison at me; now
I'm blind, I see nothing.'
He was trembling, still afraid,
on edge, as if expecting
some further blow, perhaps
the winding up of a spell.

On the examining couch
he lay supine and heard
my quiet words . . .
                                        and blinked
when my clenched fist
flashed close to his blank face.
'Did you see that?' 'See what?'
he asked, with innocence.
I murmured to myself
'Hysteria,' and smiled,
believing now that one
might cure him of his blindness.

'Keep your eyes closed
while I count up to ten:
Then open them and you will see:'
those words from my open mouth . . .
strange as an oracle!
I counted solemnly,
half dreading to reach 'ten'.
How could such magic work,
when all that I had done
was diagnose, and talk?

'Ten: open your eyes.'
He opened and cried out
'I see! I see!'
And as I touched his brow
it seemed an unsuspected power
had passed through my bones
to him—in a blinding
but sight-restoring spark that gave
new sight also to me.

EDWARD LOWBURY

Immunisation Day

Some sit pale and scared, not touching the comics,
Waiting their turn, silent and tense. They are the ones
Who know about pain, but do not cry, frozen like rabbits
In their tracks. We, the predators fill up syringes
Talking of jabs with the carelessness of a weekly chore.
Once in a while one child flies round the room, moth-like,
Screaming. We, the giants, grab him, hold him down,
And the wings fold, he is carried out, stuffed with sweets,
Sees us in his dreams at night, knocks against the trolley.
Last of all comes the survivor, who bares his own arm,
And when it's over says with distaste and severe honesty
'You hurt me. That bloody hurt, that did', We recognize
The others, but he disconcerts us, and he kicks the door
As he goes out, leaving a mark like a scratch on white skin.

ELIZABETH BARTLETT

To a Child of Five Years Old

Fairest flower, all flowers excelling,
  Which in Milton's page we see;
Flowers of Eve's embowered dwelling
  Are, my fair one, types of thee.

Mark, my Polly, how the roses
  Emulate thy damask cheek;
How the bud its sweets discloses—
  Buds thy opening bloom bespeak.

Lilies are by plain direction
  Emblems of a double kind;
Emblems of thy fair complexion,
  Emblems of thy fairer mind.

But, dear girl, both flowers and beauty
  Blossom, fade, and die away;
Then pursue good sense and duty,
  Evergreens! which ne'er decay.

NATHANIEL COTTON

A Child's Pulse

I felt the sweet child's pulse—
It sparkled like a brook.
Its source a distant heart yet it took
But little time for so many cells
To blush his rosy cheek.

It was so quick and soft—
He wanted to journey himself through the veins
That carried his blood down and aloft
Through all these hushed and curtained tufts
Back to the chambered skeins.

Here he could sing: "I am now alone,
I like your music, heart—
But I mustn't stay, I have to start
My journey all over again
To thrill your arteries and veins—"

I felt his father's pulse—he was old,
His artery so hard, so cold,
And wriggled like a snake.
I wondered had he told
His son: "I shall sleep, sleep when you wake."

HENRY SHORE

Sir of the C Stream

Old Chalky face
Mr. Teacher Sir,
hair like an unwiped blackboard
is screaming down the
endless dark corridors

"You're just a load of clots
I'd like to wash my hands of the lot of you"

He is haunted by the C stream stare
the one each backrow inherits
He knows it.
It is the ghost nailed up
behind his own eyes

A desperate inkblot of a child
how he'd struggled over the backrow corpses
the drowning and the half-drowned
treading down the clinging tendrils
of shabby family

Qualifications
                    lengthened his name
and shortened his hair
He moved to the other side of the road
where the gardens were fenced
His children said Grace
before and after meals

and then
longing for the A's the Alphas
the bright shining life-boys
he'd been allocated the C stream

"But I got out of it
I can't go through it again!" he cried
to the pins on his chair
the C stream stare
the hide and seek snigger of fingers
holding on
to the edge
of the edge

He made his desk an island fortress
bristling with shouts and canes
but his drowned child self
bobbed up and down like an Adam's apple
there was no dry land.

"I got through the exams! I did it!" he'd scream
on a cold friday afternoon
when the answers were all wrong
and there was no gleam of life

"Are you all dead at 14?"

At 14,
Old Chalky-face,
where have you been?
By 12 the little fish
are drowning in the C stream.

Have you looked in the underwater staffrooms
heard the watery roars of the half-drowned
the "made me the man I am" men
who think they've survived their childhood flood.

Wash your hands of the C stream?
Why,
it's you.
It sticks to your blood.

VALERIE SINASON

A Music Lesson

(A therapy class for brain-damaged children)

These are not ordinary children. Remote,
they sit here in a mental world that holds them
utterly still: not a foot moves, not an eye.

They listen with intent beyond the normal.
This is their genius: to compose their silence
by a mystic rule. A harpsichord

played quietly and plainly, and a prelude
uncompromising and unstopping
as the falling rain,

yet they listen out an hour's recital: taut
on their chairs, twelve children with no mind
to hint at boredom. Their shadow thoughts

drift to a high window in their head
that cannot open; happiness their instinct
draws perfunctorily from outside.

Less even than animals can they imagine
meaning Words waft past them uselessly,
but the music becomes their being:

it beats to their pulses: they are careful of its feel;
it is beauty, in its colour, order, wholeness.
It is almost language. They nearly respond.

ANN WARD

Life-Style

Promptly along the wave-length'd air
The sum of each day's woe
Invades the ear.
We pass the marmalade. The terror rising
In the throats of sixty spastic children,
As their coach begins its plunge
Into the icy waters of an Alpine lake,
Prohibits niceties of conversation.

By the time the sixtieth hand has,
For the sixtieth time, clutched
In a final, unco-ordinated spasm
At the receding air,
A shaft of sun
Illuminates the window-sill chrysanthemums.
Brown petals, unobserved, explode
Into a brazen blaze.
Pleasure, akin to pain,
Downs the drowned children.

JENNY MORGAN

But her Eyes spoke another Language

The door opened.
She walked towards the waiting seat.
She sat.
Her hands wrestled in her lap,
She crooked her fingers to conceal the nicotine stains and bitten nails,
She chewed the inner side of her lower lip,
She plucked at the clasp of her handbag,
"I have a cold," she said
But her eyes spoke another language.
"No, no trouble at home."
She flinched before the subtle onslaught,
She danced and weaved through the questions,
She ran from the truth,
She fell.
Tears welled and filled her eyes.
The comforting arm went unnoticed.
The hell she lived erupted from her lips.
She discharged herself and her shoulders crumpled.
She sobbed to a halt and dried her eyes upon a paper handkerchief.
"Thank you," she whispered and left by the back door.

WILLIAM DUNCAN

Friend at a Drug Clinic

Your steps are twisted
because your ruined city
of dark walls untouched
by the light of love has
choked your once delicate
eyes of summer seasons
with knitting, gripping,
shivering dark wards which
have soaked you with the
knowledge of death and now
through your wet eyes even
summer looks like winter.

JOHN GONZALEZ

‘This is a room like all the rest’

X-Ray

Here we see the delicate white curve of the hip,
bone meeting bone in such fragile-seeming structure,
arch and span of a human body, all flesh stripped
and dissolved in the bland dark, under the red eye,
in a moment of fear and lost dignity.

Already the machine has achieved
what the grave will do more slowly.
Already upon the mounded earth lie grieved
messages, tied to withering flowers among
the scattered dead. In this room
we see only the bright architectural square,
and the pale distribution of miniature tombs,
the dermoid cyst with its teeth and hair,
held in a shadowy void between hip and breast.

This is a life. She sees the hands
of the young Jew, and feels the cold embrace
of the cassette, and all that life has been so far
is the damp leaves in the school grounds,
and old magazines in endless doctors waiting rooms,
Sir Lancelot among the reeds, and the sweet sounds
of a badly played flute one summer evening
in Lowndes Square.

We may perceive the endless succession
of barren years, but she will always
be waiting for the flute to sound again,
and the promise to be fulfilled.

ELIZABETH BARTLETT

X Ray

Some prowl sea-beds, some hurtle to a star
and, mother, some obsessed turn over every stone
or open graves to let that starlight in.
There are men who would open anything.

Harvey, the circulation of the blood,
and Freud, the circulation of our dreams,
pried honourably and honoured are
like all explorers. Men who'd open men

And those others, mother, with diseases
like great streets named after them: Addison,
Parkinson, Hodgkin—physicians who'd arrive
fast and first on any sour death-bed scene.

I am their slowcoach colleague—half afraid,
incurious. As a boy it was so: you know how
my small hand never teased to pieces
an alarm clock or flensed a perished mouse.

And this larger hand's the same. It stretches now
out from a white sleeve to hold up, mother,
your X ray to the glowing screen. My eyes look
but don't want to, I still don't want to know.

DANNIE ABSE

The Cave

Pain is the cutting edge, the skim of a wave
Heading and pointing the rush of life,
Breaking on an unwavering cliff
Until a great cave
Is slit and hollowed into the stone.
There, but not for long,
We sit and wallow all alone.
Then we ask others to come along
To share our tearful mysteries.
But best we like to visit our neighbours' seas,
Watch them weep white
Tears down a steep stalactite,
And pile them up again in tiers.
And when the stone gleams in the borrowed light
We hold it like a shell to our ears
To hear its plight.

HENRY SHORE

The Emergency Room

This is a room no different from the rest

Look how the motes of dust dance in the sun
but lift a corner of its past
and see men running, hear their gasp
as here they meet oblivion

And I have seen the limbs deformed
crushed, twisted by the grind of steel
"fix up the drip," the order goes
and minutes more are given the soul

Life enters, life recedes as eyes
observe heart's flutter on the screen

A hand is laid on palpitating
muscle, quiet, motionless, apart

It cries and sighs within the pining creed
of twenty centuries of healing deed

Not always do they fail; at times
the overshadowing of death is baulked
and glory lights their troubled minds

But talk no more of good or ill;
of these this Lazar room knows nought

Four walls as innocent to caress
the swimmer's arms as drowned man's breast
a roof to watch the overspill
of rescue on a square of earth
and floor to catch the dropping dearth
where whirlpools eddy wild with flowers
to blossom in eternal hours

This is a room like all the rest
but less than others, less and less

A tomb where men are often laid
and after three hours some are raised
but all are kissed by mercy's dress.

S. L. HENDERSON SMITH

The Suicide

Why did we not guess?
When he drank himself blind he was erasing
A world-picture which excluded him;
When he, barely a swimmer, kept on plunging
From the top diving board, he half-hoped
There would be no water to receive him;
And when his parishioners plotted secretly
To remove the sick incumbent from his living,
He was doing his best to remove himself—
And succeeded, eventually, with coal gas.

EDWARD LOWBURY

Blood Transfusion

Blood Donors This Way—the notice broods
And rudely wakes my slumbering conscience
Devoted long to slaking passion's thirst;
My blood's my life and plainest common-sense
Dictates I summon all myself to fence
Away this sentimental call and quench
My better nature; but then goes in a woman
Miniskirted, beautiful as Eve.
I enter then. We lie together on the sacrificial bench
Victims to the medical profession,
And when the session's over, quench desire
In looks of mutual love while drinking tea.
Alas! We part but who knows but the fire
Of our twin blood may mingle in life-giving harmony
In some poor Lazarus little knowing why
His body teems with strange erotic alchemy.

S. L. HENDERSON SMITH

Portrait of William Harvey

'He did delight to be in the darke, and told me he could then best contemplate.' JOHN AUBREY

In cave like Plato's Harvey saw
The moving shadows of his mind,
And with its light dispersed the blind
Imposture of tradition's law.

Darkness and light dwell in those eyes,
Whose gaze discerned the heart's intent,
The blood's benign encirclement—
And learned in darkness to be wise.

LORD RUSSELL BRAIN

'The Questionable Terrain'

Ghosts of the Living

In this small office off the corridor
I am the Home's captive audience. Past the door
The creaking population passes to its meals
And back again to the lounges where the chairs
Have hardly cooled. Particular sounds
Attendant on the effort of the slow procession
Are so familiar. The tripod's plod, and the slight
Scrape of one shoe's toe, the squeak
Like an unoiled barrow of a swivelled caliper, the regular
Heavy sniff and wheeze of one
Who surely moves by pistons with aid of steam.
Old Shout
Yesterday worked his heavy bulk
To the dining room door, to find
He had lost his teeth. Where could they be?
Lurking under a cushion, back of the bed?
Who knows? And there was his hot meal growing cold.

I close the door on their sparrow fidget and chatter,
And see them in fantasy as perhaps they really are.
Catherine,
Not humped in her wheel chair, but running like a gazelle
Down the Home Farm meadow, gold hair flying, and her eyes
As blue as a china doll's. Arthur,
Ostling and grooming, and whistling through
His own teeth, never met her. He wenched
In a different county, and only the once. Norah
Was always a solitary, destined to teach. When
Did she bend over, never to straighten again?
Skipping, larking, singing, I hear them pass,
The young buried spirits,
The ghosts, the ghosts of the living.

MAY IVIMY

Welcome

The witty scribbles of the clematis
Over the doorway reassure the new
And hopeful patient: *Cryptograms read here.*

Neophytes, enter. Everything's prepared.
The folder bears your name. Gravely, forewarned
By your GP, the specialist attends.

You enter pallid, nameless, undefined,
But skilful hands will hold, and skilful arms
Enfold, and diagnosis christen you.

And now, newborn, you know yourself. You have
A character, and fellow-countrymen.
Obsessive, epileptic, paranoid,

Whatever your affliction, now you know
What we expect of you. We have defined;
Your task is to confirm, conform, and be

The self that we decide is right for you,
That's better than the shapeless shape you bore,
However genuine, before you came.

This is the message of the clematis.

U. A. FANTHORPE

Nurse

Tall, narrow girl, with second year belt,
She stands there, long hands
Drooling from her wrists.
One wonders how
Her grafted intestinal knowledge assorts
With her woman's weekly, daily mirror mind,
And her natural
Shrewdness. Whatever shocks
She has sustained, it seems
She has absorbed them, and not
Been much conditioned.

MAY IVIMY

For Saint Peter

I have a good deal of sympathy for you, mate,
Because I reckon that, like me, you deal with the outpatients.

Now the inpatients are easy, they're cowed by the nurses
(In your case, the angels) and they know what's what in the set-up.

They know about God (in my case Dr Snow) and all His little fads,
And if there's any trouble with them, you can easily scare them rigid

Just by mentioning His name. But outpatients are different.
They bring their kids with them, for one thing, and that creates a wrong atmosphere.

They have shopping baskets, and buses to catch. They cry, or knit,
Or fall on the floor in convulsions. In fact, Saint Peter,

If you know what I mean, they haven't yet learned
How to be reverent.

U. A. FANTHORPE

The Library

I came here often
Two decades ago
In off duty hours,
Up the stone steps
Two at a time,
Through the arched doors
In to this building
Vast, vaulted, Victorian.

I came not as the old did
Looking for peace
But with youthful excitement
My eager eyes
Roved over books
Range upon range
In search of new worlds,
Philosophies old.

In night lit wards,
Did patients wonder
What rekindled the eye
Relit the cheek
Made me more gentle
Kind to the weak.

MARGARET GILLIES

The Library

The weighty volumes look important
On the great shelves of steel.
First principles—all infallible,
Are here at hand.

In the wide hall the students pore
Over their books.
Attendants spook
In mazy corridors.

Up in the archives
Close to the primal mould
There, bound in gold,
Stands the great Book of Life.

At night when all have gone,
The Head Librarian
Reads here alone
The scrappy runes.

HENRY SHORE

Job Description: Medical Records

Innocence is important, and order.
You need have no truck with the
Seamy insides of notes, where blood
And malignant growths and indelicate

Photographs wait to alarm. We like
To preserve innocence. You will
Be safe here, under the permanent
Striplighting. (Twenty-four hours cover.

Someone is always here. Our notes
Require constant company.) No
Patients, of course. The porter comes
And goes, but doesn't belong. With

His hairless satyr's grin, he knows
More than is suitable. Your conversation
Should concern football and television.
You may laugh at his dirty jokes,

But not tell any. Operations
Are not discussed here. How, by
The way, is your imagination?
Poorly, I hope. We do not encourage

Speculation in clerks. We prefer you
To think of patients not as people, but
Digits. That makes it much easier. Our system
Is terminal digit filing. If you

Are the right type for us, you will be
Unconscious of overtones. The contrasting
Weights of histories (puffy
For the truly ill, thin and clean

For childhood's greenstick fractures)
Will not concern you. You will use
The Death Book as a matter of routine.
Our shelves are tall, our files heavy. Have you

A strong back and a good head for heights?

U. A. FANTHORPE

Case Notes

We are making a map: as two lovers
stroll together, so we step
and chain by chain discover
the questionable terrain.

I the man of category, surveyor
with an eye for country:
you, evasive traveller
companion who will deceive

Given the chance—occasionally
from a simple prudence.
Really you cannot lie
to me for our rendezvous

Does not permit of inexactitude.
In conscience now, admit
you know the ending. Beside,
old and temporary friend

Consider the design, for you must lend
your colour to define
our mutual plan. In the end
we rest, each the other's man.

KENYON ALEXANDER

Turning Point

Two burning fires of love
Looked up at me from sunken sockets,
Poured from white pillows,
So unexpected
That I, a nearly-new nurse
In pink uniform, was taken off guard,
Knocked sideways
Until swelling love
Welling inside me corrected the wobble:
I hoped my eyes answered
Oh how I hoped!
The optic messengers of this middle aged man
Last year in his prime
Now a see-through of bones.

Looking back thirty years
I still hope my eyes answered sufficiently,
Recorded the innermost 'me',
Showing I understood what he was trying to say:
Cancer had killed his words,
I, a shy inarticulate girl,
Had not yet given birth to mine.

Instinct made me clasp skeleton hand,
Kiss the pale brow,
Surprisingly strong the fierce grasp
Of one so near death:
Did he sense I wonder
That for me
He was the turning point?
From then on I loved people;
I hope.

MARGARET GILLIES

In-patients

Like children, when it's sunny they behave,
Play ball-games on the grass, run the canteen
Without much obvious embezzlement,
Are regular with drugs, use no obscene
Words to alarm the matron, kick the cat
Only in private, go for jolly walks
In healthy groups, return in time for tea,
Co-operate in therapeutic talks.

Like children, when it's rainy they are bad,
Forgetful of the needs of indoor plants,
Ignore their visitors, smoke endlessly,
Confine their repartee to *won't* and *shan't,*
Form tearstained queues outside the nurses' room,
Drink gin at night, and set fire to their sheets,
Abscond, break windows, commit suicide,
Involve us in their infantile defeats.

Like parents, we don't take them seriously.
We shrug their tantrums off as children's play,
We speak to them in kindergarten tones,
Deaf to the insult under all we say.
And when they mimic adult games, and kiss,
And talk of marriage, we applaud *How nice!*
Joyfully yoking two unstable minds,
Our wedding gift a birth control device.

Like anchorites, they guard their silent cells,
Devoted to the rituals of despair.
The bloodsoaked stone walls are inviolable,
And laymen cannot penetrate to share
The vigils these abandoned saints must bear,
Who straddle the irreconcilable
Vaults of mankind in our hygienic air,
And gasp their litanies to our dry bells.

U. A. FANTHORPE

The Night Sisters

Like bats they flew night's corridors
In their black cloaks
Visiting each dim lit ward in turn,
These winged creatures of mercy,
The Night Sisters.

Wherever they momentarily lingered
Their high frequency senses
Sent out fine pulsating waves,
Invisible antennae
Feeling for trouble.

MARGARET GILLIES

Night Duty

Swinging out over the hinterland
of other's sleep
I spiral round

on my silken thread of duty.
Spider-like
in my solitary

watchfulness I gather the lines of care,
brooding over
their trusting sleep, their

unknown dreaming lands.
I spin my web
I go my rounds.

JILL THOMAS

Night Watch

The nights we spent
Watching her cross the river
Into dreams;
The stirrings—whispering into
And disturbing linen snow,
Whilst she—
Whisked into some hot desert
Lay warmed and golden on some
Burning sand.

She lay quiet, defenceless,
Peacefully drifting over
Other lands.
Young men caressed her
Half-remembered body,
Whilst she
Murmured softly to we who watched,
Thinking our cool deft hands
Were theirs.

Sometimes, her eyes opened,
Closing out these images like
Safety screens
Between acts of a play;
But I would watch over, seeing
In her stare
Orchestras re-tuning, and
The overture heralding
Her re-entry.

The nights we spent
Watching her relax and submerge
Into coma.
Coaxing her aching body away
From total submission
Into fight.
Once or twice she woke and smiled.
Our lives, thus, clung briefly
Together.

At last, she lay
In natural sleep, waking
With the day.
We smiled in recognition
Her dreams had sunk unmentioned,
Without trace.
Mine soared with fresh reward,
Spurting with impetus to another
Night watch.

PATRICIA TORRINGTON

A Beautiful Night

How lovely is the heaven of this night,
How deadly still its earth. The forest brute
Has crept into his cave, and laid himself
Where sleep has made him harmless like the lamb;
The horrid snake, his venom now forgot,
Is still and innocent as the honied flower
Under his head—and man, in whom are met
Leopard and snake—and all the gentleness
And beauty of the young lamb and the bud,
Has let his ghost out, put his thoughts aside
And lent his senses unto death himself;
Whereby the King and beggar all lie down
On straw or purple-tissue, are but bones
And air, and blood, equal to one another
And to the unborn and buried: so we go
Placing ourselves among the unconceived
And the old ghosts, wantonly, smilingly,
For sleep is fair and warm . . . .

THOMAS LOVELL BEDDOES

To Sleep

O soft embalmer of the still midnight,
Shutting, with careful fingers and benign,
Our gloom-pleased eyes, embowered from the light,
Enshaded in forgetfulness divine;
O soothest Sleep! if so it please thee, close,
In midst of this thine hymn, my willing eyes,
Or wait the amen, ere thy poppy throws
Around my bed its lulling charities;
Then save me, or the passed day will shine
Upon my pillow, breeding many woes;
Save me from curious conscience, that still lords
Its strength for darkness, burrowing like a mole;
Turn the key deftly in the oiled wards,
And seal the hushed casket of my soul.

JOHN KEATS

The Visitors

They know no more than I would how to stand
with flowers, and being men, sheepishly clutch
them, elbows stiffly bent,
as though a touch
of clothes or hand
would wither up the bloom and kill the scent.
They do not know the odd resilience of flowers.
They wait for wife's or child's visiting hours.

Shot on jets of green the tulips zoom
and weigh their stems across the corridors,
heavy and symmetric as eggs.
The visitors
need so much room
the trolleys brush the flowers or knock their legs.
They hinder the stretcher bearing one whose life
hangs in the balance. Someone else's wife.

Then for a nurse they thin to single file
and let her through to supper as though she rushed
to tend an injury.
Awkward and hushed,
they try a smile
then shift and fidget, stood without dignity
at the beck and call of junior nurse or maid,
shielding their flowers, helpless, almost afraid.

PETER DALE

Just Visiting

I walk awkwardly between the beds in row
trying to avoid the gauntlet of levelled eyes
like beggars that ask and envy me the ease
with which I take this tailored body through.

And you are one of these faces, At first
unseen, then recognised right down the ward.
Slight twitch of greeting because I would
n't like to wear that far a smile held fast.

You whine how much your cut hurts. You tell
me nurses forced you up to pack their wads
for sterilizing, made you decorate the ward's
long walls with flowers. And you quite ill.

I'm supposed to be horrified, to sympathize.
Yet nurses have to get the dressings done,
nightly have boys to lay and drinks to down
like you to make their leaving home worth this.

Sister's periods, the old and wrinkled faces
pursed on nerve-strings to the clenched lips,
hours of obedience enough to bring collapse
on hangover, and then, clearing up faeces.

And some of them have indolent golden hair.
Over there a woman is dying, the line
of used laughter hung in bands on the lean
bones. And what you say I cannot hear.

I shudder. If your eyes started to glaze
I should listen now, although it could not lead
again to lively talk, drinks, light to slide
about your belly like brandy in a glass.

Such compassion couldn't turn a grey hair
auburn, nor startle your brows. But you will live again
and the living need a little love to go on.
You can speak now. I am here.

PETER DALE

‘Eyes That Shine’

Four Things to See

A growth of alder leaves in open light
at window height.

A wire which pulsed with speech
where spiders weave where vowels would go
where there are now no syllables to flow.

A broken slate which slipped beneath
the ribbed, ridged timber rail
which now, exposed, must fail.

The hill's skyline which stays discrete
where ice has moulded it—remote, complete.

Four things to see, four thoughts to till:
an alder tree, a telegraph, an empty shed,
a silent hill.

RONALD MANN

Discovering an Island

Discovering an island
  Of blindness in one eye,
He saw at once what most
  Can't see before they die—

The audacity of Spring
  Shot through with light that came
Not from the sun, but from
  Some living inner flame;

A threat of blindness cured
  His blindness; but how long
Could this new vision last?—
  Or was the whisper wrong

Which told him such an island
  Without views must grow
To be a continent
  Filling both eyes?—and so

He clasped the miracle
  Of his discovered sight,
But saw approaching blindness
  Like a black parasite—

Till walking, in a trance,
  Down the forlorn track
Of a disused branch line
  He felt the past rush back;

Saw steam trains that used
  To make his childhood's day—
Though in his heart he knew
  No train could come that way;

Looked hard enough to see
   The islands of the blest
Or his dead ancestors—
   And knew he was possessed;

For when he shut his eyes
   Those visions did not fade,
But filled with inner light
   The slowly gathering shade:

His sight must fail, and yet
   He found one needs no eye
To see what most can't hope
   To see before they die.

EDWARD LOWBURY

Eyes

I have examined a thousand chests,
And, obviously, twice the number of lungs.
I have handled half the number of breasts
If not in love yet in the strong
Belief I was near to work divine—
Merely because of eyes that shine.

How many times have I marvelled at limbs,
At giant muscles or golden hair.
I noted their feel, their voices' chimes.
Yet it was only through eyes, I swear,
Only through eyes I ever thought:
Here is a glance, a light from God.

Rocks need no eyes to show divinity.
They are eyes themselves through which granite views
The grain of essence and infinity.
Heaven is their puzzle, clouds are their clues.
But soft man would dissolve in the brine
Of existence had he no eyes to shine.

A blind man is different—his light is trapped
Outside a tabernacle gate.
His whole body must in light be draped
And all his face become an eye of fate.
Then he can break seals and read the line
Which is divine for eyes that shine.

HENRY SHORE

Vision

'Vision', we said, hearing how things turned out
  Just as the sage predicted; 'no mere guess:
He could see through appearances and probe
  Deep to those roots from which our future springs.'

'I had a vision,' he said; 'an angel stood
  Before me in a blaze of light; a mouth
Close to my face breathed in my ear, whispered
  'The New Jerusalem'—and I woke up.'

But one, stripped of half an eye's vision,
  Says 'Lord, let me keep what's left, to enjoy
The light of common day; spare my first sight,
  And you can keep foresight and second sight.'

EDWARD LOWBURY

The Blind Man

From the dark world I tap, tap, tap,
tap—with my invisible stick. It feels
like a whisker, it sounds like a drum. Angled,
it touches where my face will be next; where
at my side, my step cannot go. I am not,
like a spider, alive at the end of my probe:
I am not condensed at the end of my stick. I can
do it like you drive a car. I am curled
in the whorl of my ear. Do you
hear what I see?

RONALD MANN

Squint

Because I'm not sure which
  of your divergent eyes
to look at when you speak,
  you cut me down to size:

  serene, remote and wise
you seem, looking two ways
  at once. First we agree—
I catch the full gaze

of your left eye: you praise
  some person I admire;
but then I see your right
  eye gazing at the fire . . .

  so those kind words were irony!
and if I try
  some other tack, you look
embarrassed, and too shy

to look me in the eye;
  but then, turning back
to your left side, I find
  I'm on the right tack.

EDWARD LOWBURY

Limpet

Deaf—I am
aware; blind,
am troubled with touch.
Between tides
I am loyal to my rock, and rigid; beaten
cannot be prised from the ledge.

I know nothing
of the invisible side of my shell; am no more aware
how my tissues fuse with the pearl
than are you
how your muscles
insert into bone.

In the air and the light
I am still: the screech and the beak shatter my shell.
In the spray of the sea
I glide; am myself,
hungrily, avidly, making a track,
glistening, into me.

I exist
to meet my feed in the turn of the tide:
I have no other purpose,
or need. My world, older than yours, will be young
when all that was yours
will have ended.

RONALD MANN

Bones

A man is flesh and blood and brittle bones

The flesh can sing or flood the day with groans,
But what of those dour sticks with jointed ends
On which his power to stand and move depends?

What of that casket round in which is found
The mask of thought, that cage where breath is caught,
That column raising him above the ground?

Such solid basket-work no joy can lend;
And yet brave flesh has not the wit to fend
The siege of age; but you poor worthless chalk,
You only still shall balk the grave's decay
And last for aye.

S. L. HENDERSON SMITH

Feet are not Funny

The chiropody instruments, laid out
impressively at the foot of the couch,
shone efficiently but were blunt
and could not cut proverbial butter,
but the patients continued to hobble
in with corns and callouses,
desperately crying for relief
from aches which shouted from their feet.

Relaxation and a kindly patter
play their part in making better
most forms of affliction known
to man, as psychologists have shown,
and none more than chiropodists' skill
need this additive, as employed by Bill
paring and slicing millimetres of skin
to a repartee of story and fun.

Cripples floated from the surgery
following Bill's paring dexterity,
telling their friends and fellows
the feeling of relief, and his stories,
but little did they realise
this miraculous, walking paradise
arose, not from tools finely honed,
but an ordinary, one-sided razor-blade.

WILLIAM LINDSAY

'No Notes to Chart our Journey'

Old Men in a Home

They don't move much. Mostly
They have dropped anchor,
Harboured in armchairs
With pedestal ashtrays
And cupsidors—
Since expectoration is not allowed
Where it is most convenient.

The curtains of age
Almost completely drawn,
They sit there singeing
Their fingers and burning holes
In the plastic urine-proof rexine,
Rolling their own, or
Ramming it into cindery bowls
Imperturbable
As rows of Sioux
And staining the ceiling.

Should one, like a maverick tom,
Encroach another's ground,
Lower his creased old worsted backside
Into another's chair,
Then senile passion flares
Into a filthy flame;
The crutch used for support
Becomes the weapon of assault,
And the old leg that cannot stand
Without the aid of stick,
Will stand, to strike the blow.

MAY IVIMY

Geriatric

She sat looking like
a ball of wool—blindfolded
with memories; unconcerned
with the encircling time
which silently captured and
carried her to the awaiting
tide of sleep.

JOHN GONZALEZ

Emergency Gastrectomy

Sent for this case, I found an executive
too overweight for one to lift alone.

I thought, awaiting help with eighteen stone,
you'll weigh far less to bring back if you live.

But later when I took him back to bed
his swag of flesh was harder still to lift.

There were blood-drip, saline and flush to shift,
three bottles to be kept above the head.

Sweating and winded, we dumped the slipping load.
I freed my arms—my hands were covered in blood.

PETER DALE

From Endymion

A thing of beauty is a joy for ever:
Its loveliness increases; it will never
Pass into nothingness; but still will keep
A bower quiet for us, and a sleep
Full of sweet dreams, and health, and quiet breathing.
Therefore, on every morrow, are we wreathing
A flowery band to bind us to the earth,
Spite of despondence, or the inhuman dearth
Of noble natures, of the gloomy days,
Of all the unhealthy and o'er-darkened ways
Made for our searching: yes, in spite of all,
Some shape of beauty moves away the pall
From our dark spirits. Such the sun, the moon,
Trees old, and young, sprouting a shady boon
For simple sheep; and such are daffodils
With the green world they live in; and clear rills
That for themselves a cooling covert make
'Gainst the hot season; the mid forest brake,
Rich with a sprinkling of fair musk-rose blooms;
And such too is the grandeur of the dooms
We have imagined for the mighty dead;
All lovely tales that we have heard or read:
An endless fountain of immortal drink,
Pouring unto us from the heaven's brink.

JOHN KEATS

Pathology of Colours

I know the colour rose, and it is lovely,
but not when it ripens in a tumour;
and healing greens, leaves and grass, so springlike,
in limbs that fester are not springlike.

I have seen red-blue tinged with hirsute mauve
in the plum-skin face of a suicide.
I have seen white, china white almost, stare
from behind the smashed windscreen of a car.

And the criminal, multi-coloured flash
of an H-bomb is no more beautiful
than an autopsy when the belly's opened—
to show cathedral windows never opened.

So in the simple blessing of a rainbow,
in the bevelled edge of a sunlit mirror,
I have seen, visible, Death's artifact
like a soldier's ribbon on a tunic tacked.

DANNIE ABSE

Hiroshima

Now the trumpet of the atomic gale
Blasts through the interstices of flesh.
Cell shakes from living cell, and the pale
Bone unknots the vapour of its mesh.
Now every monument to power
Is bared of laurels by its breath,
And all dominion in an hour
Sinks to the level entropy of death.
Is this the end? Or has one wayward spark,
Shot from the bonfire of the world's decay
Sown in some distant star the flame of birth,
Somewhere restored the loveliness of earth—
A chaffinch singing in the Milky Way,
The phoenix shining in the burning dark?

LORD RUSSELL BRAIN

The Operation

There should always be something casual
About an operation, otherwise
How could a man dare hold lancet
With intent to cure, not kill, but find
Himself careering hand in hand
With death, not his but of another
Of whom the very tendrils of substantiation
Fall through his fingers?
And that is why they chatter to distract
As do steeplejacks, from too much pressing
Matter, to pretend it lessens
Tension; it is the instruments I love
Caressed in tight-gloved fingers
Rapped against palm to fasten
Pulsing worms of artery,
Probe out disease, touch, burn and linger
And at last tie bootlace-like
Strong hoods of tissue to the wound
So that this woman be intact again
Whom they have god-like bound
With catgut that roots of pain
Crawl crab-like into her no more
But leave her manacled to mystery,
While they retire in infinite disdain.

S. L. HENDERSON SMITH

Heart Surgery

You decant his blood out
Into a machine
Prime it with artificial fluid
During the operation
Then you put it all back
Fibrin clot and platelet
So that heart brain bladder and intestines
Will be patched up

You play at being minor Gods
Put him on a foam mattress
Control his temperature
Regulate his heart
By an artificial pacemaker,
Monitor his brain function
Coagulate and necrotise
Put him back to life

My poor patient
You open your eyes
And ask "Whose dim shape do I see?"
From clouds of unconsciousness
You float out
Arms too heavy with transfusions
You feebly try to greet me
As I squeeze your lungs into the depths
Of your bronchial tree
I pillage
And suck out a beautiful cast
Fit for a museum

Your thin bony fingers
Haunt my sleep
Till the next bleep
Your faintly blue tinge
Is like my heavy lidded eye
Before I surrender again
To scientific zeal

E. MITTER

A Phantom Limb

"A patient who has lost a limb by amputation may continue to feel as if the limb were still there, and may even experience pain in the phantom limb."

Russell Brain, *Diseases of the Nervous System*

He tries to forget the crash, to erase a moment
When the Jaws, ready to receive him, fastened on
His left leg; and then, as though in answer
To prayer, sensation flickered and returned
Where once the leg had been—each toe in place,
Each tendon where it was. With eyes shut
He could regard it as a miracle,
A new leg to replace the one sawn off—
No stranger, in its way, than what a crab
Or lobster takes for granted. Moments later
Coming to his senses, he looks back and finds
The whole improbable episode a nightmare
From which he now wakes up, and the left leg—
Tingling where, so it seemed, no leg remained—
Is real and living as before the nightmare:
What happened, in that case, was not the crack
Of bones, not bleeding, disarticulation,
But laboured breathing or dyspepsia,
Or a high wind with rain slashing the windows
While he was sleeping; what on other nights
Might have promoted dreams of air attack,
Of earthquake, or of Hell . . . But this red pain,
These lightning twinges in the invisible limb
Are real as lightning: "If the pain is real,
The limb is real", he argues, drawing comfort
From what to others looks like mockery.
Delirious, like a medium he awaits
The phantom, which returns to haunt his body
With much more certainty than any ghost
Has ever haunted; wilful; sporadic;
Now absent for a while; soon changing shape;
Shrinking; dissolving; after months no more
Than a haze of pain, a reminder of the Jaws
That still require some human sacrifice.

EDWARD LOWBURY

Radium Therapy

Deflated of flesh,
like axehafts,
the shinbones poke from rumpled bedding.

I hurry past
to avoid the radiation field.
The sweat and stench would make one retch.

But turn
to put the blankets straight.
And, leaning through the field,
I warm myself a little in my haste.

PETER DALE

The Stethoscope

Through it,
over young women's abdomens tense,
I have heard the sound of creation
and, in a dead man's chest, the silence
before creation began.

Should I
pray therefore? Hold this instrument in awe
and aloft a procession of banners?
Hang this thing in the interior
of a cold, mushroom-dark church?

Should I
kneel before it, chant an apophthegm
from a small text? Mimic priest or rabbi,
the swaying noises of religious men?
Never! Yet I could praise it.

I should
by doing so celebrate my own ears,
by praising them praise speech at midnight
when men become philosophers;
laughter of the sane and insane;

night cries
of injured creatures, wide-eyed or blind;
moonlight sonatas on a needle;
lovers with doves in their throats; the wind
travelling from where it began.

DANNIE ABSE

Not Dead but Sleeping

She didn't lie long, they said,
clutching their soiled dressing gowns
to their wrinkled drooping breasts.
It was a mercy really.

There is a death in the home,
a room is vacant now, her bottles
of gin have been whisked away,
her library books returned.

The Victorian drains smell foul
in the summer time. Death
has a smell too, a cleaned room,
a disinfectant washed floor,

a nakedness, and a futile sadness,
for now it all begins again.
One by one they drop like ripe
fruit into the waiting basket.

There is a conspiracy of silence
behind the other doors, a frantic
dusting of ornaments and turning
out of drawers in the succeeding days.

On the day of the funeral the flowers
are returned from the hearse and they
pick them over, florist's flowers
jammed into unsuitable vases.

This is her legacy; an odour
of carnations, which masks the smell
of drains as it also masks
the fear of who goes next.

At night the lights go out
one by one as they lay alone,
waiting for the hand to shake
the branch in the invisible air.

They don't sleep well. Reaching
out to the commode they stumble
and clutch at a chair, or make
a warming cup of tea,

to pass the dawdling hours
before the dawn comes up
and they can hear the milkman
leaving a pint at the wrong door.

Silly bastard, they think, rattling
their walking frames in impotent rage,
he doesn't know she's passed away.
Nobody thought to tell him—

she is not dead but sleeping.

ELIZABETH BARTLETT

Woman in the Hospital for Incurables

She has refused injections to kill pain;
they are too painful, she protests, for her fleshless body,
confusing them with the more difficult hurt
of dying alone. Crossing the heath I visit her,
tactlessly with mud on my boots and the glow of wind.
We speak of travel and music and the never-coming spring.
One dying in unnecessary pain
in the unpeopled night
will not cry for the lost grass and irretrievable music.

DAPHNE GLOAG

Sexual Delinquent

We are all keen to take a look at him.
Women from other departments find excuses
To come into the room
And see what he looks like.
What have we all imagined?
Some hairy hero
Bulging with sex and muscles?
Some sleek seducer,
With an irresistible moustache and
A smooth line in sales talk?
Or even our own boyfriend,
Improved a little, given that keen interest
In women that so few men
Really have?

But all we see
Is a pale, lank-haired pilferer,
Hungry for food, love, anything available,
In charge of a capable spinster.

U. A. FANTHORPE

Music in a Dark Room

We listen to Debussy with the lights turned off.
The fire is warm and the day's quota of suffering
is over, and we think we are happy for the length
of a disc, for a space in time where the ear is all,
where there are no words, only notes in the fall
of the light rain mingling with his recurring
bell sounds.

The old, the sick, the dying, the spina-bifida child,
the malingerers and the manic-depressives, at once
so wild, so quiet, according to the swing of the disease,
go away for this short, short time. This dark room
rings and trembles, fades, washes like limpid waves,
restores and comforts, renews and revives us,
for we need it, and so will they, in us, tomorrow.

ELIZABETH BARTLETT

A Mood

I want a holiday
From medicine and death
To the arts
I always read poetry with alternating
pages of anatomy
Listen to Fabrizio
Morimmo a stento
Before every viva
I want to paint trees
Tall and splendid
Reaching up to the sky
To some destination
Unlike myself
The afternoon sunlight of a snowy winter
Catches all the picture of loved ones
And lights up their eyes and smiles and deeds
And shines from the copper of the fireplace
As I listen to madrigals
On this New' Year's afternoon

E. MITTER

Consultant's Holiday

His enemies: death, suicide, the slow
Phlegmatic non-existence of despair,
Obsession's endless wood of private fears.

His soldiers: bored, promiscuous, with low
Morale and bad feet, not the type to share
Heroic vigils on the mind's frontiers.

His weapons: therapy of various sorts,
Drugs, treatment, hobbies, even work. Such arms
Sometimes explode, and injure his own men.

His allies: friendly tribes, whose dullness thwarts
Elaborate manoeuvres with alarms
Of missing cats, or time for tea again.

His leave's spent fighting on a different front,
Tracking down distance, loneliness and cold
In their Scots fastness. These he traps and kills,

But when time's up, returns to his own hunt,
To find his side demoralised and old,
Despair and death glowing like daffodils.

U. A. FANTHORPE

Physician, Heal Thyself

I find you tousled in a bed
Of clothes, living your own graph
Victim not victor now, not judge
But pleading plaintiff for your life;
The sound of hearts, your bread and meat
Now echoes drum-beats of your own;
All men must one day take
Medicine they make for others,
Authors written, painters
Portrayed, parsons prayed upon;
I stroke the white soft of your flesh
May hem-virtue of your own
Not work physicians' alchemy?
As I turn to go, I know
A hundred spirits wait
To will you benefit of clergy;
One last look, how like a bird
You are, the healing gone, the wings
All spent a patient aeon since
At someone else's heaven's gate.

S. L. HENDERSON SMITH

Patients

Not the official ones, who have been
Diagnosed and made tidy. They are
The better sort of patient.

They know the answers to the difficult
Questions on the admission sheet
About religion, next of kin, sex.

They know the rules. The printed ones
In the *Guide for Patients*, about why we prefer
No smoking, the correct postal address;

Also the real ones, like the precise quota
Of servility each doctor expects,
When to have fits, and where to die.

These are not true patients. They know
Their way around, they present the right
Symptoms. But what can be done for us,

The undiagnosed? What drugs
Will help our Matron, whose cats are
Her old black husband and her young black son?

Who will prescribe for our nurses, fatally
Addicted to idleness and tea? What therapy
Will relieve our Psychiatrist of his lust

For young slim girls, who prudently
Pretend to his excitement, though age
Has freckled his hands and his breath smells old?

How to comfort our Director through his
Terminal distress, as he babbles of
Football and virility, trembling in sunlight?

There is no cure for us. O, if only
We could cherish our bizarre behaviour
With accurate clinical pity. But there are no

Notes to chart our journey, no one
Has even stamped CONFIDENTIAL or *Not to be*
Taken out of the hospital on our lives.

U. A. FANTHORPE

Pantomime Diseases

When the fat Prince french-kissed Sleeping Beauty
her eyelids opened wide. She heard applause,
the photographer's shout, wedding guest laughter.
Poor girl—she married the Prince out of duty
and suffered insomnia ever after.

The lies of Once-upon-a-Time appal.
Cinderella seeing white mice grow into horses
shrank to the wall—an event so ominous
she didn't go to the Armed Forces Ball
but phoned up Alcoholics Anonymous.

Snow White suffered from profound anaemia;
the genie warned, 'Aladdin you'll go blind,'
when the little lad gleefully rubbed his lamp;
the Babes in the Wood died of pneumonia;
D. Whittington turned back because of cramp.

And schoolmaster Jack, behind the sheds, caressed
schoolgirl Jill, one third his age and pantless.
Then, panting, they went up the hill and back
till Cupid's leaden arrow in his chest
caused a flutter, a major heart attack.

When the three Darling children thought they'd fly
to Never-Never Land—the usual trip—
their pin-point pupils betrayed addiction;
and not hooked by Captain Hook but by
that ponce, Peter Pan! All the rest is fiction.

DANNIE ABSE

‘They all, still, smile like that’

Tied under my Heart

A little slice of humanity,
tied under my heart,
I offered you
the right to reality.

A next-to-nothing piece of girl,
silenced by the womb,
you spoke to me
of perpetuity.

Summer grows cold in my hands
but everywhere
the beginnings of life
clamour
and I can smell the sky
moving over to morning
on the weasel-early wind.

And one day you will fly,
my fledgling daughter,
proud and unconquered,
from day to day to day.

JUDITH SMALLSHAW

The Obstetrician

A piece of blank paper
Is a uterine lining,
Clean.
No sperm, no ova.

The poet's task
Is to implant
Sperm and ova
Both at once.

An embryo
Needs cells galore.
A poem only
A cell or two.

Watch head or breech!
Heed nature's course,
And tamper
Only if you must.

HENRY SHORE

The Knife

A steady hand, a scalpel's fluent stroke:
Taut skin and flesh were quickly laid aside—
The blade cut deep, the uterine muscle broke
To burst the bubbling amniotic tide.
And from the spewing of the drenching flood,
Just like a hand drawn from a soiled, split glove,
A child was lifted, whelped in pain and blood:
The living, breathing aftermath of love.

JUDITH SMALLSHAW

Birth

Christ I said aloud.
I was animal,
my body drowning me with birth.
It was all of all time
in the red of the over early morning.

My blood froze in my head
making a quiet thunder.
I was awake to the huge tearing,
the concrete hurt—
solid and shocking.
I cried into the pillow:
light minded with fear,
afraid to die.

And this time I couldn't run away.

Look down, they said,
and see.
But my body wept, tight-eyed,
and held its breath
for the coming of this suckling legacy
from love.

JUDITH SMALLSHAW

The Mountaineers

Climbing their way through their maternity,
At steeper gradients they rest awhile
And ponder every step their Herculean task,
Prepare for last assault, and summit reached
They sit and stare, at all the beauty lying there
And wrap the sun, the moon, the stars
Round the small bundle in their arms.

CHRISTINE BRESS

The Smile Was

One thing I waited for always
after the shouting
after the palaver
the perineum stretched to pain
the parched voice of the midwife
          Push! Push!
and I can't and the rank
sweet smell of the gas
and
          I can't
as she whiffed cotton wool
inside her head
as the hollow stones of gas
dragged
        her
            down
from the lights above
to the river-bed, to the real stones.
          Push! Push!
as she floated up again
muscles tensed, to the electric
till the little head was crowned;
and I shall wait again
for the affirmation.

For it is such:
that effulgent, tender, satisfied
smile of a woman
who, for the first time,
hears the child crying the world
for the very first time.

That agreeable, radiant smile—
no man can smile it
no man can paint it
as it develops without fail,
after the gross, physical, knotted,
granular, bloody endeavour.
  Such a pure spirituality, from all that!

It occupies the face
and commands it.
            Out of relief
you say, reasonably thinking of the reasonable,
swinging, lightness of any reprieve,
the joy of it, almost helium in the head.

            So wouldn't you?
And truly there's always the torture of the unknown.
There's always the dream of pregnant women,
blood of the monster in the blood of the child;
and we all know of generations lost
like words faded on a stone,
of minds blank or wild with genetic mud.
            And couldn't you
smile like that?

Not like that, no, never,
not with such indefinable
dulcitude as that.
And so she smiles
with eyes as brown as a dog's
or eyes blue-mad as a doll's
it makes no odds
whore, beauty, or bitch,
it makes no odds,
illimitable chaste happiness
in that smile
as new life-in-the-world
for the first time cries the world.
No man can smile like that.

2
No man can paint it.
Da Vinci sought it out
yet was far, far, hopelessly.
Leonardo, you only made
Mona Lisa look six months gone!

I remember the smile of the Indian.
I told him
            Fine, finished,
you are cured
and he sat there smiling sadly.
Any painter could paint it
the smile of a man resigned
saying
            Thank you, doctor,
you have been kind
and then, as in melodrama,
            How long
have I to live?
The Indian smiling, resigned,
all the fatalism of the East.
So one starts again, also smiling,
            All is well
you are well, you are cured.
And the Indian still smiling
his assignations with death
still shaking his head, resigned.
            Thank you
for telling me the truth, doctor.
Two months? Three months?

And beginning again
   and again
whatever I said, thumping the table,
however much I reassured him
the more he smiled the conspiratorial
smile of a damned, doomed man.

Now a woman, a lady, a whore,
a bitch, a beauty, whatever,
   the child's face crumpled
as she becomes the mother,
she smiles differently, ineffably.

3
As different as
the smile of my colleague,
his eyes reveal it,
his ambiguous assignations,
good man, good surgeon,
whose smile arrives of its own accord
  from nowhere
like flies to a dead thing
when he makes the first incision.

Who draws a line of blood
across the soft, white flesh
as if something beneath,
desiring violence, had beckoned him;
who draws a ritual wound,
a calculated wound,
to heal—to heal,
but still a wound—
good man, good surgeon,
his smile as luxuriant
as the smile of Peter Lorre.

So is the smile of my colleague,
the smile of a man
secretive behind the mask.

The smile of war.

But the smile, the smile
of the new mother,
what
        an extraordinary
          open thing
                it is.

4
Walking home tonight I saw
an ordinary occurrence
hardly worth remarking on:
an unhinged star, a streaking gas,
and I thought how lovely
destruction is when it is far.

Ruined it slid
on the dead dark towards fiction:
its lit world disappeared
phut, through one punched hole or another,
slipped unseen down the back of the sky
into another time.

Never,
not for one single death
can I forget we die with the dead,
and the world dies with us;
yet
in one, lonely,
small child's birth
all the tall dead rise
to break the crust of the imperative earth.

No wonder the mother smiles
a wonder like that,
a lady, a whore, a bitch, a beauty.
Eve smiled like that
when she heard Seth cry out Abel's dark,
earth dark, the first dark
eeling on the deep sea-bed,
struggling on the real stones.
Hecuba, Cleopatra, Lucretia Borgia,
Annette Vallon smiled like that.

They all, still, smile like that,
when the child first whimpers like a seagull
the ancient smile reasserts itself
instinct with a return
so outrageous and so shameless;
the smile the smile
always the same
                    an uncaging
                      a freedom.

DANNIE ABSE

'If there are Ghosts to raise'

EMILY DICKINSON—in appreciation

A broken heart does best
in a well-appointed room,
with knick-knacks here and there
and a discrete rose in bloom:
calamities of heart and sense
befit pretence.

ROY BATT

Dream-Pedlary

If there were dreams to sell,
  What would you buy?
Some cost a passing bell;
  Some a light sigh,
That shakes from Life's fresh crown
Only a rose-leaf down.
If there were dreams to sell,
Merry and sad to tell,
And the crier rung the bell,
  What would you buy?

A cottage lone and still,
  With bowers nigh,
Shadowy, my woes to still,
  Until I die.
Such pearl from Life's fresh crown
Fain would I shake me down.
Were dreams to have at will,
This would best heal my ill,
  This would I buy.

But there were dreams to sell
  Ill didst thou buy;
Life is a dream, they tell,
  Waking, to die.
Dreaming a dream to prize,
Is wishing ghosts to rise;
And if I had the spell
To call the buried, well,
  Which one would I?

If there are ghosts to raise,
  What shall I call,
Out of hell's murky haze,
  Heaven's blue pall?
Raise my loved long-lost boy
To lead me to his joy—
There are no ghosts to raise;
Out of death lead no ways:
  Vain is the call.

Know'st thou not ghosts to sue?
  No love thou hast.
Else lie, as I will do,
  And breathe thy last.
So out of Life's fresh crown
Fall like a rose-leaf down.
Thus are the ghosts to woo;
Thus are all dreams made true,
  Ever to last!

THOMAS LOVELL BEDDOES

Evocations

By dream or blood transfusion they are recovered
deceitful and mooning from the doubtful region,
careless in the detail of body: the best
part of them stays there.

They come with reluctance, but the white eyes shift
down slowly to focus in air and they look
knowing, murmur quiet enigmas, smile or
simply ignore us.

Their noses peak and sparkle with sweat; sometimes they
crowd long gangplanks to a quay in gas-bleached
uniforms, explaining the larger wounds to
all who will listen.

Of course there are distinctions: the dream-dead go back,
follow their dim callings elsewhere, while patients
in time pencil newspaper margins, making
maps of the journey.

But if by our charity the drip is stopped?
A quiet statement then gapes from the bed and the dry tongue
foretells an untimely return: in this case
differences vanish.

KENYON ALEXANDER

Looking for Something?

Always puzzled, the man I keep seeing
Who charges down the road, stops, turns,
Runs backs, stoops to pick up something,
Throws it down, turns again, stoops,
Picks up something, throws it down, runs . . .

Always alone, he looks as much lost
As what he is looking for; will stop to think
While crossing a road of screaming brakes. A ghost,
He scares off neighbours who might help. Louts
Laugh at the man, shout 'Look, the missing link!'

More puzzled than upset, he never speaks
To passers-by, never complains; but sometimes
Growls at baiting boys, spits, shakes
A helpless fist, and then goes on scanning
Gutters, pavements, other people's homes.

I'd like to help—but has he really lost
Anything? When I catch his eye, a look
So vacuous meets mine, I see, at last,
He is seeking something he has never had,
And has no clue what it is, or what it's like.

EDWARD LOWBURY

Know Yourself

What am I? how produced? and for what end?
Whence drew I being? to what period tend?
Am I the abandoned orphan of blind chance,
Dropped by wild atoms in disordered dance?
Or from an endless chain of causes wrought?
And of unthinking substance, born with thought?
By motion which began without a cause,
Supremely wise, without design or laws.
Am I but what I seem, mere flesh and blood;
A branching channel, with a mazy flood?
The purple stream that through my vessels glides,
Dull and unconscious flows like common tides:
The pipes through which the circling juices stray,
Are not that thinking I, no more than they:
This frame, compacted, with transcendent skill,
Of moving joints obedient to my will;
Nursed from the fruitful glebe, like yonder tree,
Waxes and wastes; I call it mine, not me:
New matter still the mouldering mass sustains,
The mansion changed, the tenant still remains:
And from the fleeting stream repaired by food,
Distinct, as is the swimmer from the flood.
What am I then? sure, of a nobler birth.
Thy parent's right I own, O mother earth;
But claim superior lineage by my Sire,
Who warmed the unthinking clod with heavenly fire:
Essence divine, with lifeless clay allayed,
By double nature, double instinct swayed,
With look erect, I dart my longing eye,
Seem winged to part, and gain my native sky;
I strive to mount, but strive, alas! in vain,
Tied to this massy globe with magic chain.
Now with swift thought I range from pole to pole,
View worlds around their flaming centres roll:
What steady powers their endless motions guide,
Through the same trackless paths of boundless void!

I trace the blazing comet's fiery trail,
And weigh the whirling planets in a scale;
Those godlike thoughts, while eager I pursue,
Some glittering trifle offered to my view,
A gnat, an insect, of the meanest kind,
Erase the new-born image from my mind;
Some beastly want, craving, importunate,
Vile as the grinning mastiffs at my gate,
Calls off from heavenly truth this reasoning me,
And tells me I'm a brute as much as he.

JOHN ARBUTHNOT

The Maze

They understood each other well.
Up there the sungod in his golden rooms,
and below, brutality prowling the sewers.

So many seekers! Not only the Athenian boy
with his ribbon, who stabbed so earnestly
and boasted a rare return to light,

but all others who must hunt down corridors
for the ceaseless bellow of anguish, stumbling
till they perish in their maze.

The beast? A twitching, massive, horned head
swivelling murderously, with blood on cheek
or faceless, as your history decides.

He shambles close, yet so nearly invisible,
the eyes glowing black in the hot dark, that men
speak of the labyrinth called Minotaur.

And who may tell the heart of the matter?
Perhaps there is always a central, legendary dread,
and round it, corner pointing to corner,
the unfinished web of loss, the catacombs of pain.

NORMAN KREITMAN

Cavatina

Didn't you notice
there were angels around
in the art room today.
Didn't you see the anxious faces
of those coming into the room?
Then a cup of coffee
or dark brown tea
from the aluminium pot
sipped slowly to the sound of the guitar.

Then talk—talk of good moments
our peak experiences
and the handling of the music box
with the toy dancer
bewitching the child in us,
like when we blew bubbles on Thursday last.

Didn't you notice
the angels arriving
and the faces changing
smoothing and smiling
while we and the angels listened
to John Williams playing a cavatina.

PATRICIA BALL

The Angel Collector

I know a man
Who collects angels.
Just as some collect
Stamps
And butterflies—
He collects angels.

In a large red room
In boxes lined with velvet,
Under glass,
Chests pierced
With swords,
They sparkle in the light.

At night
One can hear their whirring
Wings beat at the glass,
For they are still alive—
The collector in his bed
Smiles.

I once asked the man:
"How do you catch angels?
What time, what season?"
"With a net" he said.
"At midnight
And in summer."

I had always thought
He was a man,
But now I feel uncertain:
He looks so strange,
And limps
On his left foot.

HENRY SHORE

Electroencephalogram

'Now I'm going to give you a perm', she says;
clipping the sleek electrodes smartly in,
rigging the open face with rubber tubes,
checking the nerve-white leads back
to the steel box.

And world lies back, wondering
whose brainwave this is, what the sheet will show:
closing its eyes to chance, leaving its waking fate
to eight pens on an impassive tide
of smooth paper scribbling soundlessly, decisively . . .

eight pens in a calm or choppy humour
plotting nothing or its sinister equivalents:
the whiff of sea-mist drifting dizzily across,
the foam and crumple of compulsive epilepsy,
or the slouched rock of some inoperable tumour

pressing on to an incredible catastrophe
like murder, say . . .
all predicted in this weather-girl's bleak witchcraft;
graph of a skull that could be hung, one day,—
now drawn and quartered in advance.

GEOFFREY HOLLOWAY

The Visitors

'This patient was obviously hallucinating as I spoke to her'—
Consultant's note.

There was one in the room, thinking of the sherry
he would have before lunch, rocking slightly in his chair.

There was another, opposite him, grey hair falling
across her face, like a coy but ravaged schoolgirl.

There were others present to whom she would have talked
had he not asked her tedious questions, eyeing her.

They were invisible to him, his ego balanced well,
his libido functioning perfectly, his accountant satisfied.

Sometimes their faces got between her and the desk,
mocking and sullen, whispering foul insinuations.

When they advanced too fast across the carpet
she wanted to get up and tell them to go away,

but his tight clinical voice held her rigidly poised
between the overt grins and the beckoning hands.

In the end, he won, and the others bobbed like balloons
in a corner, unmistakably there, but further away.

She was compelled to tell them to go right away from her
though she could see them reflected in his glasses, waiting.

As he asked her questions, he noted down her hesitant
answers in a precise hand on a long yellow form.

In the end, he formally escorted her out into the corridor;
the faces, mouthing obscenities, followed in a muddled bunch,

crowding with her through the narrow door, accompanying
her back to the ward where they settled in like squatters,

one on the end of the bed, some by the locker,
and one who laid his head on her pillow, talking softly

until she fell asleep abruptly, and for a while
the visitors crept away silently, or floated out

leaving only the faintest trace of their presence,
like a perfume, or a discarded cigarette burning away.

ELIZABETH BARTLETT

Therapy

Touching the well-springs
Releasing the silt of years
That the waters of life
May flow and revive
The flower.

PATRICIA BALL

Ode on Melancholy

No, no, go not to Lethe, neither twist
Wolf's-bane, tight-rooted, for its poisonous wine;
Nor suffer thy pale forehead to be kissed
By nightshade, ruby grape of Proserpine;
Make not your rosary of yew-berries,
Nor let the beetle, nor the death-moth be
Your mournful Psyche, nor the downy owl
A partner in your sorrow's mysteries;
For shade to shade will come too drowsily,
And drown the wakeful anguish of the soul.

But when the melancholy fit shall fall
Sudden from heaven like a weeping cloud,
That fosters the droop-headed flowers all,
And hides the green hill in an April shroud;
Then glut thy sorrow on a morning rose,
Or on the rainbow of the salt sand-wave,
Or on the wealth of globèd peonies;
Or if thy mistress some rich anger shows,
Emprison her soft hand, and let her rave,
And feed deep, deep upon her peerless eyes.

She dwells with Beauty—Beauty that must die;
And Joy, whose hand is ever at his lips
Bidding adieu; and aching Pleasure nigh,
Turning to poison while the bee-mouth sips;
Ay, in the very temple of Delight
Veiled Melancholy has her sovran shrine,
Though seen of none save him whose strenuous tongue
Can burst Joy's grape against his palate fine;
His soul shall taste the sadness of her might,
And be among her cloudy trophies hung.

JOHN KEATS

Schizophrenia

If anyone comes, asking if I am here,
Tell them I have gone away.

I have gone into no voices for the speaking with,
Under gargoyles with ears for all hearing with,
Wet with streaked tears for no weeping with,
And cannot come when you call
With your high voices through the wall,
You changing people, grown large, grown small
For my torment.

If a man comes, bearing golden apples,
Tell him I will have none.

I have no use for apples not for the eating of,
Or a heart rigid for the loving with,
My mouth is not for kissing, but for grimacing with,
And my stained clothes will never be for the cleaning of.
Your hands lift me up and out of my bed,
Your white starch rustle-talks
For my torment.

If a woman comes, holding a child by the hand,
Tell her it is not mine.

I have a hollow which is not for the filling of,
And breasts which have no hope for the sucking from,
And a demon who is not for the killing of.
I am alone for the loneliest dream there is dreaming of.
Your drugs are white grit in my mouth,
For my poisoning, for my dying of,
For my torment.

But if a child comes alone with an armful of toys,
Tell her I am here in my bed.

Her doll is for my clasping and my talking to,
And her puppets for my playing and fondling of,
Her giants and her dead princesses for my looking at,
Her birth for my death, on a sheet for the winding-in,
Her silence for my psaltery of laughter,
No dirtier and no dafter
Than I ever was.

ELIZABETH BARTLETT

We are all a little Mad

"The man is mad", they said,
"He claims to have moonlight
Locked in a shell, and he
Will not eat, sleep or even
Make love; for he fears that
Should he remove his hands
The light would escape".

Yes, the man was mad and we
The nurses in our snowwhite
Coats took the shell and
Smiled, but I being a poet
Had to look inside and as I
Did, the man smiled and said,
"It's gone".

JOHN GONZALEZ

'No Room for False Emotion Here'

Don't Call

Reporting on my friend after his fall—
  This message from the Intensive Care Unit:
    'Deeply unconscious . . . On a respirator . . .
we'll call you when we want you here . . . Don't call.'

A foregone conclusion. When they said
  'His brain has died; may we switch off the breather?'
    We had no option; but a streak of guilt
Surprised us, as we murmured: 'What is 'dead'?'

And then, weeks after his burial,
  I dreamt the telephone was ringing; he
    was on the line, his voice far off, half-drowned
By crackling, but I heard him say: 'Don't call.'

EDWARD LOWBURY

Congers

First Autumn leaf: predictable, still, sad;
opaque, full of its shape, not knowing
the vivid, green lawn. The yellow dead leaf,
and the living green lawn, touch and oppose.

I am not wanting to write of that leaf's death
or the coming of Autumn.

                                        This morning,
at the railway crossing, I watched the train recede:
a long straight line, the hills distant;
the black guard's van becoming grey, minuscule,
filled up with distance. Most things recede, fade,
elude our understanding.

                                        What it is in our lives
is not in our dimension.

RONALD MANN

The Destroyers

I know where the destroyers live:
In forests of gold
Swaying heavy emerald branches.
Here the destroyers lay in wait,
Here the great lover,
The youth of the cross without jewels,
Passed by on his evening walk
Dreaming of his mother's eyes.

They hacked coral wounds
Deep in his sacred flesh.
Ambulances rushed,
Surgeons in silver theatres
Sewed his wounds with threads of gold,
Dusted them with diamond.
But they must fester
Waiting for the unction of love.

HENRY SHORE

Poem in the Mirror

The irony of personal loss
blots out a universe of pain.

Hold to such an hour. It is
the mirror of the naked soul

revealing bone and hunger unadorned
behind whatever face a man might proffer.

And as the world ticks again into motion,
mechanical, steel-grey before the shoots

of the new and acid Spring emerge,
hold yet within the ear

the cry of the wolf baying in winter
for all he has lost, and cannot find.

NORMAN KREITMAN

Franco

Drugs made his belly
break and bleed;
drawing the surgeon's scalpel
to kill the physician's wrong.
Dialysis
changed his poisoned blood,
the intricate coils
charging his life.
Anti-coagulants
pitched their tents
in his thrombosed veins.

But had they the right,
that regiment
of self important people,
to keep the poor old man
half alive
so long?

How dared they play
at being God?
Could they dictate
whether he was to live
or when he was to die?
Viva España!

Doddering and drooling
he may have been,
his once proud heart unmindful
of his boasting youth.
But would you endure it all
for two more weeks
of tenuous old age?

He had lived his lifetime,
never mind the blind side
of his politics—
he was still human:
and we are all everyman.

Death could have come
with dignity . . .
or was the thunder of the Vatican
too loud?

JUDITH SMALLSHAW

Emily Drowned

She asked me, aching-eyed.
I nodded. She sighed.
A twenty second silence followed,
Intense, explosive, hollowed
From the echo of the vaulted ceiling,
Charged with growing feeling.
"Oh! no, Oh! no," she screamed and sank her nails into her husband's shoulder.
He, not much older,
Comforted her in vain
And stemmed his agony with a taut drawn rein.

A policeman came in haunting blue.
I left the parents to their loneliness and walked out through the hall. In the street
My feet
Threw shattering steps upon the tar. We stopped. The officer lifted the tailgate
Of his van and I heard him grate
His teeth. There, lying on a tartan rug lay
Emily—three yesterday—
Pale and cold, she unmoving, I so moved that I nearly cried.
I had to touch her skin to certify her death.
I raised her eyelids. My misted breath
Dulled the already dull complexion of her eyes. She was dead.
I nodded to the officer. "She's dead," I said
And thought of my own small daughter
Asleep at home in bed. Emily had drowned in two feet of water in the field behind
Her house. The weather signed
The sadness of the evening
With a bereaving
Winter shower.

I had to return to the parents who would sob for hour
On hour in each other's arms.
Gone were the infant charms
That dressed their home,
They cried together, but, alone.

WILLIAM DUNCAN

Time To Kill

Even now, Hippocrates, you can't restore
A lost soul to the battered skull, or stop
This maniac frenzy of the wrong cells
That multiply like a deranged computer.

You've had more luck with other spells: with germs
That melt the flesh, but melt away themselves
Under the magic of a secret code—
Until they solve the code, and then return.

You will try anything—a change of skin;
A change of heart, even; now there's talk
That you have found a way of beating Death—
Letting the heart, at least, go on and on:

Rare for the favoured few (if they stay sane),
This moonshot in a world of traffic jams!
But if the gamble really works, and Death
Goes under—so, it seems, go Love, and Birth.

The suffering stretch out their hands and beg:
"Preserve our lives"; the best you ever do
Is to prolong them; whether or not the germ
Is burned out, Death scores in the end—

And just as well; you'd have to invent some drug
To cure a man of immortality,
If it should come to that, and re-instate
The Old Man's Friend, the Young Man's Advocate.

EDWARD LOWBURY

Old Age of a Clown

In a way, it's more pathetic than the dotage
  Of scholar, poet, statesman,
For this one never seemed to age—
  Or, for that matter, to grow up;

A permanent child, he kept us laughing through
  Five decades; when we walked, he ran,
Or hopped, or capered—yet he knew
  Some day such larks would have to stop.

Translated at one stroke from infancy
  To old age, the jester seems
To have by-passed maturity.
  And staggers, puzzled, through his dreams.

EDWARD LOWBURY

On a Death in an Old People's Home

(To the memory of Elizabeth Williams)

I was busy, with the normal course of events,
Telephoning, actually, when they told me
"Willie's gone." A muscle in my heart
Contracted, pinched the blood,
In my throat a frog swelled.

Inevitably, with us, death
Like tea, has its routine;
The doctor, the mortician, the next of kin
Play their part in the disposal, and must be notified.

I wandered down the corridor,
Made empty by Willie's going,
A picture of the daughter in my eyes.
Pale, delicate skin, the auburn hair
Her mother's, but young and gleaming,
The soft brown eyes shattered, like pools
Whipped up by the wind, and the water spilled.

She's already taken
Some of life's punishment—
Her husband's unskilled wage,
Three small boys ambitious
For bicycles and trips with the school abroad,
And the bruising sequence of 'flu, washing, measles, shopping—
And Mum—

Her kind heart become an organ fighting
To maintain the paralytic frame,
Her capable hands deprived
Of all refined movement, her speech
Distorted and uncontrolled, with dribbling tongue;
And still behind the grotesque disabilities—
Mum—

The mind unharmed, the simple qualities
Of kindness, humour, love, all evident.
Willie would toddle about, a bit too fat
For her heart, and give a hand
To the more infirm; a simple joke
Would shake her frame with laughter,

A touch of trouble, in one of her letters perhaps,
Or another old lady poorly, and she would weep
With an infantile bellow and baby tears.

I could not bear
Willie to cry.
I would cradle her in my arms and beg her
Not to cry, in desperation
I would make her laugh (she laughed so easily).
I was afraid those tears, that heaving fleshy bosom,
Would release the damned-up sorrows
Of all humanity.

I found her on her bed, the nurse
Removing pinafore, dress, stockings—
Sitting in her armchair she'd mercifully
Slipped away unknowing. I asked to help, and soon
The pale, naked body lay there, still
Limp and warm, the face calm and slowly
Smoothing out—only the hands
And fore-arms very cold. I cradled the head
For the pillow to be straightened, the grey hair patched
With flaming auburn, and wisps of nasturtium wool
Still flaring on the fair skin
Of the innocent body. Surely never

Did a body die, though limited
By low estate, tethered
To poverty all her life,
Surely never
Did one die more pure?

In the kitchen, near, a girl
Student domestic, working vacation, sobbed
Her sorrow for Willie, all her tears
Streaming along her long, long dark hair, like a flood
Of black sorrow. Suddenly,
My hand on the young bony shoulder,
Willie's hair
Burst out like a flame somewhere.

MAY IVIMY

The Layer-Out

There is no loveliness in death

The drooling mouth falls open
And blood contained a lifetime's breadth
Falls moaning from the coping stones
Lonely as an abandoned fool

How merciful the cotton wool
The prayer-book underneath the chin
The woman

This is a task that suits a woman best
Who knows love's grotesque aftermath;
A man can never enter in
This emptiness; he rests and sleeps;
It is the woman keeps her path of sin
And clothes the seed with ironed linen
Anointed, clean.

S. L. HENDERSON SMITH

Post Mortem

How strange that for a little span
A clod should look so like a man!

Intent on utterance unheard
Appear so wise, yet speak no word;

Unthinking wear the mask of thought,
Submit to all, but suffer nought,

And bear on an impassive face
The sculpture of a secret peace!

LORD RUSSELL BRAIN

Post-Mortem

Detached always detached,
No room for false emotion here;
Any such thoughts would leave the door unlatched
And hinder science; the doctor's heart must always fear
The unguarded catching of the throat,
The pang of love, remorse, or any passion
Which siren-like, might rock the fragile boat
Of steely self-control tradition-fashioned
Wherein he floats.

These organs were my friend's,
My patient's rather; so who wins?
How can I know where mortal body ends
And laughter, shared joys' power,
The riddle men call soul begins?

He died you say of this and that;
I guessed as much so now let's close the story,
How comforting to know the answer pat;
But I emerge and still the hidden glory
Of mystery-laden depths unplumbed assails me
As transitory once-relied-on compass points recede
And thoughts stretch out horizon-wards
Insatiate as the sea.

S. L. HENDERSON SMITH

On Edmund Burke

Here lies our good Edmund, whose genius was such,
We scarcely can praise it or blame it too much;
Who, born for the universe, narrowed his mind,
And to party gave up what was meant for mankind;
Though fraught with all learning, yet straining his throat
To persuade Tommy Townshend to lend him a vote;
Who, too deep for his hearers, still went on refining,
And thought of convincing, while they thought of dining;
Though equal to all things, for all things unfit;
Too nice for a statesman, too proud for a wit;
For a patriot, too cool; for a drudge, disobedient;
And too fond of the *right* to pursue the *expedient;*
In short, 'twas his fate, unemployed or in place, sir,
To eat mutton cold and cut blocks with a razor.

OLIVER GOLDSMITH

Epitaph on Colonel Francis Chartres

HERE continueth to rot
The body of FRANCIS CHARTRES:
Who, with an INFLEXIBLE CONSTANCY and
INIMITABLE UNIFORMITY of life, PERSISTED,
In spite of AGE and INFIRMITIES,
In the practice of EVERY HUMAN VICE,
Excepting PRODIGALITY and HYPOCRISY:
His insatiable AVARICE exempted him from the first,
His matchless IMPUDENCE from the second.

Nor was he more singular in the undeviating *pravity of his manners,* than successful in *accumulating* WEALTH:
For, without TRADE or PROFESSION.
Without TRUST of PUBLICK MONEY,
And without BRIBEWORTHY SERVICE,
He acquired, or more properly created,
A MINISTERIAL ESTATE.

He was the only person of his time
Who could CHEAT without the mask of HONESTY,
Retain his primeval MEANNESS when possessed of
TEN THOUSAND a year;
And, having daily deserved the GIBBET for what he *did,*
Was at last condemned to it for what he *could* not *do.*

O indignant reader!
Think not his life useless to mankind!
PROVIDENCE connived at his execrable designs,
To give after-ages a conspicuous proof and
EXAMPLE
Of how small estimation is EXORBITANT WEALTH
In the sight of GOD, by his bestowing it on the
most UNWORTHY OF ALL MORTALS.

JOHN ARBUTHNOT

John Donne speaks from his Grave

At last within my tomb I lie.
Pity me not, O, passer-by!
Since Death and I in life were one,
I cannot be by Death undone.

When every other pleasure flies,
Death's a delight that never dies.
In his perpetual dower house
The worm, my widow, is my spouse.

No more need I reproach the sun,
That all too soon the day's begun.
Descend, eternal night, and hide
The cold caresses of my bride!

LORD RUSSELL BRAIN

Resurrection Song

Thread the nerves through the right holes,
Get out of my bones, you wormy souls.
Shut up my stomach, the ribs are full:
Muscles be steady and ready to pull.
Heart and artery merrily shake
And eyelid go up, for we're ready to wake—
His eye must be brighter—one more rub!
And pull up the nostrils! his nose was snub.

THOMAS LOVELL BEDDOES

The World of Light

They are all gone into the world of light!
  And I alone sit lingering here;
Their very memory is fair and bright,
  And my sad thoughts doth clear.

I see them walking in an air of glory,
  Whose light doth trample on my days:
My days, which are at best but dull and hoary,
  Mere glimmerings and decays.

O holy Hope! and high Humility,
  High as the heavens above!
These are your walks, and you have showed them me,
  To kindle my cold love . . .

If a star were confined into a tomb,
  Her captive flames must needs burn there;
But when the hand that locked her up gives room,
  She'll shine through all the sphere.

O Father of eternal life, and all
  Created glories under Thee!
Resume Thy spirit from this world of thrall
  Into true liberty.

Either disperse these mists, which blot and fill
  My perspective still as they pass:
Or else remove me hence unto that hill
  Where I shall need no glass.

HENRY VAUGHAN

In Winter, Elms

Each of these twigs of tree
has stretched and flexed
to gain most space:
the trunk divides,
thick branches writhe,
twigs interlace—
so must events have changed.

This elm, whose symmetry is etched,
whose twigs display their fan through space,
tells history; chimes out,
beside the stone-white tower,
gargoyles of moments when the wet wind came,
the seasons changed, when one long growth
obscured the next—
and so, both changed.

Branches now bend to shape events which were
when they were half their length,
one-third their width,
one-tenth their strength—
now they are old and strong
and neither flex, nor bend,
nor fill with throstle's song.

RONALD MANN

'The Healer Walks with Burning Hands'

Fire-Mass

When the fire-Mass over London was being said,
The elevation was the Sun and the whole thing
A body of broken rubble by the River Thames,
Lit up with fire and fingering searchlights. Once,
Spattered by falling stone, I froze in an archway,
And two girls were standing there. They said nothing,
But I could see the taller and more attractive,
Restless with her fingers, and the other, conscious of me,
Not wanting to interfere in my desire to touch her friend.
What comfort in a kiss there is I do not know.
Over the shoulder of the tall girl, while we kissed,
My eyes uncovered the relieved face of her friend.
The foul night-dust changed easily to day;
And it was spring, and death was streets away.

RUSSELL GRANT

Unconscious Woman

Perhaps this day the sun may waken her,
Split wide the cocoon of hard sleep,
Draw her out into a changed time.

She will emerge,
Bedraggled as a damp insect;
Knowing fear again.

She will realize herself,
Be aware of her transfiguration,
Live again in the coil of the senses.

She will sip at the reviving nectar
Of the spirit, touch again the texture
Of life. Butterfly woman, taste each hour.

JILL THOMAS

Elms in Winter

Elms in Winter: when the leaves are down
  An untrained eye can see
    No difference between dead wood and living:
    A black, inverted lightning
  Frozen to permanence, each leafless tree,
Dead or alive, towers bravely on the skyline.

Odd that such skeletons should be alive!
  Imagine a graveyard
    Where, in the Spring, some femur sprouted flesh
    While others showed no change;
  Telling which are the living would be hard:
A solid ghost might step from any grave!

Taking this road in June, I looked away
  From the pandemic shock
    Of sick and ravaged boles. To-day they seem
    Less bleak; look much the same
  As those which, having shed their foliage, mock
The dead, like spiders waiting for their prey.

These elms, riding the snow in mock death,
  Are living skeletons;
    Knowing the Spring that's in their bones, we see
    Even the dead tree
  As if caught in suspended animation,
All set once more for the routine rebirth.

EDWARD LOWBURY

Learning to Breathe

I've been learning to breathe under water. Don't laugh.
The flood level has already risen overhead and is
still rising. It doesn't leave much time.

Of course, I'm not the only one to be submerged. Several
of my best friends have already drowned. They sway here
and there as the eddies carry them. I try not to look.

Gradually the lungs fill up and it begins to seep into
the circulation. The crucial moment! Don't think it
won't flow in your arteries. Only too easily!

Concentrate rather on one cell in your brain. Keep that
dry. To try to save the whole brain at once . . . you'll
only end up by drowning. With one synapse, even one
cell, it's quite possible to survive.

I'm learning to breathe but it's slow work. As of today,
I can breathe perhaps twice, or if I'm lucky, three
times a month.

This may seem a negligible accomplishment. But then,
perhaps the flood level hasn't risen so high in
your part of the world, as yet.

GAEL TURNBULL

The Homecoming

There were great birds circling.
Clearly the portents were all awry, the hour perturbed.
From the city breathless messengers began to arrive,
choking with news, and the shouting drew nearer.

But his wife sat with her maid, in tranquility,
even when the shrubs were trampled down
by the hubbub of neighbours.

Lazarus stood in the doorway: eyes met
in silence. Uneasy, he drifted to the table
prepared elaborately against his homecoming,
but the bread had only the known taste of death.

Why had he returned? Once his beloved has deeply grieved,
and revived, and lifted her head to breathe again
—that man stays dead for ever.

NORMAN KREITMAN

Faster than Light

"At last I seem to need no time for any journey;
 Fixing my thoughts upon that star from which the light
Travelled six thousand years to reach me, I am there
 At once. . ." the old man muses, lets me share

Such thoughts, dragging his feet beside me down the Causeway;
 "Your Concordes and Apollos deafen, but they're slow;
To reach my destination I break the light barrier—
 In silence, too; no-one will notice when I go."

Listening, I found myself translated to his language.
 Already he had put his clock into reverse,
Taking me with him on a jaunt back to the beginning—
 No passport needed there, and the route might have been worse.

Did he realise, when we stopped in the cold night to receive
 Orion or the multipoint injection of Pleiades,
What was to follow—the explosion that carried him away
 To his real destination? There was no time to grieve.

Faster than light? perhaps the question has no meaning;
 He was moving now—if 'moving' is the right word—in
A dimension through which light can't penetrate. Nothing
 Can move faster than light, and now he too was nothing.

EDWARD LOWBURY

Renewal

Where the bomb fell,
The shattered trees from broken boughs
Put out fresh leaves;
And August, when already
The dry leaf scrapes along the pavement,
August sees, delicately green,
The tender promise of a second spring.

So may the broken life
Break into leaf again;
Suffering renewal, like a tree
Hiding its grief among new branches,
Finding itself once more
Shaped after its kind, restored.

LORD RUSSELL BRAIN

A Visit to the Zoo for the First Kidney Transplant Mothers and their Children

The camels might never have been here.
They stand tall and indifferent
while the children climb between their humps.
The government minister holds a baby; mothers
are almost blooming and carefree. They own the day.
"Minister, Minister," shout the photographers,
"look this way please." Camels dying
in deserts are far and forgotten nearly.

Beyond the zoo wind tangles
in precarious grass, temporary daffodils
are suddenly remarkable. This day of camels,
warm camel breath, the ugly convenient humps
are irreplaceable. A moon-faced mother,
amused, absorbed, holds up her child
to the camel's brown, comfortable hair,
straggling, undeniable.

DAPHNE GLOAG

Baby Giraffe

I have never seen
anything more beautiful
than that baby giraffe
at the Zoo.

String thin, gangling,
wobbly standing,
big big brown eyes,
eyelashes thick silk sticks,
outshining film stars,
Young, vulnerable,
as all young are.

That is why, when you,
sit desolate, unhelpable,
I talk about the baby giraffe
that day at the zoo.
I say what I believe,
who thought up that giraffe
thought up you.
Life is not meaningless
with baby giraffes at the zoo
and you.

PATRICIA BALL

At Jesty's Tomb

(for Bryan Brooke)

Benjamin Jesty (1746-1816), a Dorset farmer, is described on his gravestone as "the first person (known) that introduced the cowpox by inoculation and who from his strength of mind made the experiment from the cow to his wife and two sons in the year 1774." This was 24 years before the first published account (by Edward Jenner) of vaccination against smallpox.

Few, of course, could take it seriously,
  That claim of yours to cast the devil out
In single combat, without sorcery—
  Or prayer, even; there was truth, no doubt,
In how you explained it: that you had the aid
  Of friendlier fiends; not witchcraft? even if
Your claims were true, should one not be afraid
  To shield those who, through sin, must come to grief?
Wise after the event, immune to pox
  And ballyhoo, we shake our heads and smile:
Such rot! but now the devil's on the rocks
  And reason is in charge—at least, while
Our vaccines work and there's no plague to fear.
You've had the last laugh, old pioneer!

EDWARD LOWBURY

After the Dark Months

The sunlight seems fragile,
the blackbird in the angle of the tree
seems vulnerable, the walking of the birds
under the tree, among the leaves,
splinters of sunlight and shadow, seems
too delicate to last.

Quick, quick they move and cross the road,
their backs iridescent—shining like the waxed,
sun-glittered leaves of Spring.

The bark of the beech is smooth
on this warm day in which the sunlight,
for the first time since the dark months,
is bright enough
to make the potted plant
upon the window ledge
transparent with green light.

It is not meaningless—
but tragic,
hidden.

RONALD MANN

The Dyke

I have met a fortunate few
Who have never been aware that it existed;
That it stood, safely encircling their lives.
They have managed to survive, their certainties intact,
Their skies as blue as when they were first fathomed.

Taken for granted, like health and husbands,
You only notice it when the first breach appears.
The black waters enter, trickling in rivulets
And patterning the land with dark threads
Or, as the case may be, crashing across the walls,
Breaking them down and covering the fields.

When the tide ebbs, as all tides must,
The dyke will be re-built, as all dykes must
Or, as the case may be, simply patched up.
The salt mud must be made fertile.
In time, with work, or alternatively,
Without appearing to bother very much,
New grasses grow—even a few trees.

It will not happen again. The dyke is stronger,
Built to withstand further destruction.
The builder knows his apple trees will bloom;
That in the autumn fruit will appear and fall
Just as it did before, only the taste
Will have altered.
And in blossom time it will be necessary
To view the flowers from a different perspective.

JENNY MORGAN

A Spastic Child on a Pony

Bodily bewildered
Michael
sits a horse;

rolling, reeling,
restless
as yes and no,

his happiness hugs
his odd
and awkward face.

From his saddled
refuge
he screams out

his toothy pleasure
to his
half-way brain.

This now-time is the
heart's-ease
of his week:

Nohow so snug
as in
his walking sleep

when he can run
and shout
like other boys—

but somehow it is
almost
second best.

JUDITH SMALLSHAW

To Sir Charles Sherrington

On his 90th birthday

Man shapes the patterns of his mind
As models of the world without,
But to himself he long was blind
And found no answer to his doubt.

You first within the brain discerned
The meaning of its ordered ways,
And man of his own nature learned
To thread the labyrinthine maze.

Poet, you saw the vibrant nerves
Subdued to metrical control,
By which each one in rhythm serves
The guiding purpose of the whole.

These lines a homelier homage bring
Than all the laurels time has brought—
A wish as birthday offering
From world-wide children of your thought.

May age, which clouds the body's eye,
Still leave undimmed the inward sight
That reads life's secret poetry
With timeless wonder and delight!

LORD RUSSELL BRAIN

Success in Malaria Research

This day relenting God
  Hath placed within my hand
A wondrous thing; and God
  Be praised. At his command,

Seeking His secret deeds
  With tears and toiling breath,
I find thy cunning seeds,
  O million-murdering Death.

I know this little thing
  A myriad men will save.
O Death, where is thy sting?
  Thy victory, O Grave?

SIR RONALD ROSS, written 1897

To One Who Has Been Long in City Pent

To one who has been long in city pent,
'Tis very sweet to look into the fair
And open face of heaven—to breathe a prayer
Full in the smile of the blue firmament.
Who is more happy, when, with heart's content,
Fatigued he sinks into some pleasant lair
Of wavy grass, and reads a debonair
And gentle tale of love and languishment?
Returning home at evening, with an ear
Catching the notes of Philomel—an eye
Watching the sailing cloudlet's bright career,
He mourns that day so soon has glided by:
E'en like the passage of an angel's tear
That falls through the clear ether silently.

JOHN KEATS

Recovery

Impossible to tell
    at first,
if in the final count
    it will be ill or well
with them.
    If the slim hand
lying inert
    on the coverlet
will surmount
    that sudden, grievous hurt.

Her eyes besought, 'How soon
    will you know
when, if ever,
    I shall again
hold a bow,
    and begin to sweep
exultant joy or deep
    impassioned sorrow
from a violin?'

When at last she firmly trod
    the floor
and gripped my hand,
    when reflexes once more
were instant and complete
    and she became aware,
fully to realise
    she was all right;
the radiance in her eyes
    was so intense,
I swear
    I saw the hand of God
switch on the light.

JULIE BALL

Walking by the Sea

They feel the calm delight, and thus proceed
Through the green lane—then linger in the mead—
Stray o'er the heath in all its purple bloom—
And pluck the blossom where the wild bees hum;
Then through the broomy bound with ease they pass
And press the sandy sheep-walk's slender grass,
Where dwarfish flowers among the gorse are spread,
And the lamb browses by the linnet's bed;
Then 'cross the bounding brook they make their way
O'er its rough bridge— and there behold the bay!—
The ocean smiling to the fervid sun—
The waves that faintly fall and slowly run—
The ships at distance and the boats at hand;
And now they walk upon the sea-side sand,
Counting the number and what kind they be,
Ships softly sinking in the sleepy sea;
Now arm in arm, now parted, they behold
The glittering waters on the shingles rolled;
The timid girls, half dreading their design,
Dip the small foot in the retarded brine,
And search for crimson weeds, which spreading flow,
Or lie like pictures on the sand below;
With all those bright red pebbles that the sun
Through the small waves so softly shines upon;
And those live lucid jellies which the eye
Delights to trace as they swim glittering by:
Pearl-shells and rubied star-fish they admire,
And will arrange above the parlour-fire.

GEORGE CRABBE

St. Luke's Little Summer

October. The sumach sheds crimson light
  As though it sensed a black presence
Waiting in the wings. Prompted, the tree
  Makes the most of summer's brief renascence;

We'd like to keep such things for good. The leaves
  Ooze a light redder than roses,
Fluorescent, a sunset glory;
  But then, before the spotlit scene closes,

The boughs shed leaves—at the least puff
  Dozens fall just when they're given
Earthly perfection—or perhaps
  Have trespassed to a foretaste of heaven.

Having shed light, then leaves, the tree becomes
  A skeleton. We may console
Ourselves, though; like a spider
  It's aping death; fierce buds wait on the bole.

St. Luke, revered physician, you'll delight
  In your short summer, and the news
Of the cured sun: the blood flows
  More freely, making us love before we lose.

EDWARD LOWBURY

Deliverance

The healer walks with burning hands.
Spines straighten, knots melt.
And death is humble, understands.

Moving to his bright commands
nothing is that is not felt.
The healer walks with burning hands.

Blind eyes have found their suns,
lost ears their singing quilt.
And death is humble, understands.

The crutch is sloughed, the cripple runs—
past buried, future built.
The healer walks with burning hands.

Love is the least of his demands,
faith what his fingertips have smelt.
And death is humble, understands.

Flame without fear has crossed the lands,
poor have danced, tyrants knelt.
The healer walks with burning hands,
and death is humble, understands.

GEOFFREY HOLLOWAY

Index of Authors

The Contributors

DANNIE ABSE had his first book of poems published while still a medical student at Westminster Hospital, London. After qualifying in 1950 he continued to write professionally and every five years or so has had a book of poems published. His *Collected Poems 1948–1976* was published by Hutchinson in 1977. In 1973–74 he was writer-in-residence at Princeton University, then returned to work as a chest specialist in London. He is well known for two outstanding autobiographical books, *Ash on a Young Man's Sleeve* and *A Poet in the Family* and quite recently Robson Books published *My Medical School* which Abse edited and which contained autobiographical pieces by eminent doctors. His two most recent plays, *Pythagoras* and *Gone in January*, have been produced at the Birmingham Rep. and at the Young Vic Theatre in London. He is the editor of the annual *Best of the Poetry Year* (Robson Books), a selection of prose and poetry from the magazines published in Britain.

KENYON ALEXANDER. Born 1921. Educated at Birkenhead School and Liverpool University, from which he graduated MB, ChB in 1944. Served in RAMC in India. Trained in pathology at Cambridge and since 1955 has practised as a consultant pathologist (latterly specialising in haematology) in South Warwickshire. He began writing poetry in 1970, when he shared first prize in the Stroud Poetry Festival.

JOHN ARBUTHNOT (1667–1735). Graduate of St. Andrews, became Physician Extraordinary to Queen Anne, and was a member of the literary circle which included Pope and Swift. He wrote both pamphlets and medical works. Pope's Prologue to his *Satires* is addressed to Arbuthnot.

JOHN ARMSTRONG (1709–1779). Armstrong took his degree of MD at Edinburgh and practised as a physician. Wrote *The Art of Preserving Health*. Author of a satirical poem, entitled *Taste*.

JULIE BALL was born in St John's Wood, London, and educated at various schools, both private and within the state system. After working as a Civil Servant for a time, she was for several years secretary to a General Practitioner. Her final appointment before retirement was to the post of Cardiographer at Sutton Hospital. Her *A Dash of Angostura*, a collection of poems, was published in 1978 by Outposts Publications.

PATRICIA BALL. Born London 1912. Educated in Public Libraries, but compelled to spend precious time in state schools. Art training at St Albans' School of Art and two years Jungian analysis for Art Therapist post at Hill End Hospital, St. Albans. Edited two poetry anthologies, *The Shattered Heart* and *Song in a Strange Land*.

ELIZABETH BARTLETT. Born in Deal, Kent. Educated at State schools. Secretary/Receptionist to a General Practitioner for the last ten years, but now under the National Health Service on call for the Home Care Service at week-ends. Her poems have appeared in *Outposts*, *The New Review*, *Tribune*, *Poetry Review* and the P.E.N. and Arts Council anthologies. Her first book of poems, *A Lifetime of Dying* (Peterloo Poets) appeared in 1979.

ROY BATT. Born London 1934. Graduated as a Veterinary Surgeon—Liverpool 1958; in Anatomy (Medical School, Liverpool) 1960; and as Doctor of Philosophy—Reading 1974. During the 60s and 70s he lectured and researched in universities. Research interest has been chiefly in an inherited illness in animals, similar to one in children. This involved working for a year at Los Angeles Hospital (1972–3). He is at present Lecturer in Anatomy at the Royal Veterinary College, London.

THOMAS LOVELL BEDDOES (1803–1849) went abroad to study medicine and lived in Zurich after 1835. Although his most important work, *Death's Jest Book*, was commenced in 1825, it was not published until 1850, after his death by suicide.

LORD RUSSELL BRAIN (1895–1966) Walter Russell Brain was born at Reading. Educated at Mill Hill and New College, Oxford, but left Oxford after a year to join the Friends Ambulance Unit and was made orderly to the X-Ray Department. He was transferred to the FAU at Jordans and then drafted with a company to the King George Hospital, London (in the X-Ray Department once again). Here he met Stella Langdon-Down, whose grandfather and father were distinguished physicians, and she encouraged him to take up medicine. So he started evening classes at Birkbeck College, in zoology, botany, physics and chemistry, and passed both the conjoint and the London MB in these subjects. In 1919 he went back to New College as a medical student and passed in June for the Oxford BM. He took a war degree on his first BM in anatomy and physiology, being awarded the Theodore Williams Scholarship in physiology. Won the Southern and Andrew Clark Scholarships and qualified BM, BCh (Oxon) in 1922. Then followed a variety of appointments at Maida Vale Hospital, The London, Moorfields, Mount Vernon, and the Infants Hospital, Vincent Square. It would be impossible to do justice to his contributions in the medical field and interested readers are referred to the Royal Society's Biography. His *Poems and Verses* was privately published in 1962. He received many honours. He was knighted in 1952, became a baronet in 1954, and was created a Baron in 1962. Elected FRS in 1964.

CHRISTINE BRESS. Born at Falmouth, 1920. Daughter of a Methodist Minister. Educated at Kent College, Folkestone. Eight years nursing experience in hospitals, plus varied work since in many fields. Considerable experience in dealing with both the mentally and physically handicapped. At present running an antique shop. Hobbies: writing, painting, travelling. Her work has been featured in several anthologies, and Outposts Publications published her first collection of poems, *The Think Tank*.

NATHANIEL COTTON (1705–1788) studied medicine at Leyden and followed the profession of physician. He was Keeper of a Lunatic Asylum for a time, where Cowper was an inmate. A volume of his collected poems was published in 1791.

ABRAHAM COWLEY (1618–1667) was born in London and educated at Westminster School and Trinity College, Cambridge. His *The Mistress*, published in 1647, brought him recognition as one of the leading poets of his time. During the civil wars he supported the royal cause and went into exile with Queen Henrietta Maria in 1646. Returned to England in 1656 and took his MD at Oxford.

GEORGE CRABBE (1754–1822). Born at Aldeburgh and mainly self-taught. Apprenticed to a doctor and later practised medicine himself. Took orders in 1781 and was appointed chaplain to the Duke of Rutland from 1782 to 1785, and subsequently served the community as a clergyman, with an absorbing interest in literature and botany. His *The Village* appeared in 1783, *The Parish Register* in 1807 and *The Borough* in 1810.

PETER DALE was born in 1938, and educated at Strode's School, Egham, and St Peter's College, Oxford. Before going up, he worked for two years in hospitals, first at St Peter's Hospital, Chertsey as a theatre porter, and then in the Radcliffe Informary as a general porter. The experience of these years went into the poems of the *Rooted in Earth* section of his Selected Poems, *Mortal Fire*, from which the poems used here are taken. His most recent books are the Penguin translation of the selected poems of Villon and a sonnet sequence *One Another*, published in 1978 by Carcanet and Agenda Editions. At the moment he is Head of English at Hinchley Wood School, Esher, and the Associate Editor of the quarterly *Agenda*.

WILLIAM DUNCAN (William Duncan Bright Darbishire). Born 1946 in the English Lake District. Educated locally. Married 1969, two children. 1965–70 Liverpool Medical School (MB, ChB 1970), 1970–73 Hospital posts in Southport and Kendal, 1974 onwards Family Doctor in Ulverston, Cumbria MRCGP).

U. A. FANTHORPE was born in Kent, educated in Surrey and at Oxford, and taught English at Cheltenham for 16 years. Then broke away from the system and tried various temporary jobs. She is now working as a clerk in a Bristol Hospital. Her first collection, *Side Effects*, was published by Harry Chambers in the Peterloo Series, 1978.

SIR SAMUEL GARTH (1661–1719) was born in Yorkshire and educated at Ingleton School, Peterhouse (Cambridge) and at Leyden where he read medicine. Elected a Fellow of the College of Physicians and practised as a physician. Member of the Kit-Cat Club. His satire, *The Dispensary*, published in 1699, was an attack upon the opponents to the proposals for a dispensary for the poor. A friend of Alexander Pope who described him as "the best good Christian without knowing it." Subsequently appointed Physician General to the army and Physician in Ordinary to George 1.

MARGARET GILLIES was born of Scottish parents and brought up in Scotland. She started training as a nurse at 18 at the Dundee Royal Infirmary in the early 1950s. Worked in Surgical, Medical, Children's and ENT Wards, also in the theatre. Is a State Registered Nurse. Worked for six months in an Out-patients Clinic and then married a farmer. Has seven children. Lived three years in Canada. Started writing poetry seriously about four years ago.

DAPHNE GLOAG lives in Hampstead. She read Classics and Philosophy at Somerville College, Oxford, and after a short spell of teaching worked for the Medical Research Council for many years, largely on publications. She is now a staff writer with the *British Medical Journal*, and the poems in this volume were prompted by her work there. Her poetry has been published in magazines and anthologies and broadcast.

OLIVER GOLDSMITH (1728–1774). Son of an Irish parson, Goldsmith graduated BA at Trinity College, Dublin. Studied medicine at Edinburgh and Leyden and is said to have obtained a degree in medicine in Europe. Returned to London in 1756 and had difficulty in supporting himself as a physician, as an usher, and as a hack writer. Friend of Samuel Johnson. His best known works are the novel *The Vicar of Wakefield* (1766), the play *She Stoops to Conquer* (1773) and *The Deserted Village* (1769).

JOHN GONZALEZ was born in Gibraltar in 1946, but has lived in Britain since 1954. After working at various jobs, on leaving school at the age of 15, he spent three years as a novice in a nursing order in Ireland. On his return to England he worked in a Geriatric Ward for almost three years and then commenced training, subsequently serving on an Orthopaedic and Geriatric Ward. He is shortly due to commence training again for Mental Handicap Nursing.

RUSSELL GRANT was born in 1924. Graduated in medicine at Glasgow University and started General Practice in Chelsea in 1952. Spent a year in Paris and Italy, writing. Took up psychiatry at the Maudsley Hospital in 1954, and did two years research in the psychiatry of children in Canada (published in 1956–57). Subsequently has been Principal in General Practice at King's Cross, having helped to set up the Government hostel for homeless women, in what he calls The University of St. Pancras.

GEOFFREY HOLLOWAY spent six years in the Royal Army Medical Corps, working with the Field Ambulance, General Hospital and the Parachute Field Ambulance, as Nursing Orderly and as post-operative Nurse in surgical teams. Then two years as a social worker in a psychiatric hospital and twenty years as a mental health worker with Westmorland County Council. As a poet he has contributed widely to literary periodicals and anthologies, and has had three volumes of poetry published.

MAY IVIMY. For many years worked for Hertfordshire C.C. Department of Social Services in Homes for the Elderly, having contact in the early days with tramps, vagrants and homeless families, as well as with problem elderly and senile cases. She has seen great changes in the Social Services from the converted workhouses and reception centres for "gentlemen of the road" to the present day purpose-built Homes, where single bedrooms are the rule and a happy, positive approach to the clients prevails. Her poems have appeared in many journals and anthologies. Her *Night is Another World* was published by Outposts Publications in 1964, and *Midway this Path* in 1966, when she won the Manifold Chapbook Competition. A member of the Executive Council of the Poetry Society from 1966 to 1973. She has been Editor and Organiser of Ver Poets since its foundation in 1966, and on the Council of the Society of Women Writers and Journalists, with special regard to poetry, since 1975.

JOHN KEATS (1795–1821) was the son of a livery-stable keeper. He was apprenticed to an Edmonton apothecary, but his indentures were cancelled in order that he might qualify as a surgeon. Although passing his examinations, he abandoned surgery for literature. Shelley assisted him to publish *Poems by John Keats* in 1817 but it was not a financial success. In the year that he wrote *Endymion* he nursed his brother, Tom, until he died. In 1819 wrote *The Eve of St Agnes, La Belle Dame Sans Merci, On a Grecian Urn, To a Nightingale, To Autumn,* and *On Melancholy.* Seriously ill with consumption, he left England for Italy in September 1820 and died at Rome the following year.

NORMAN KREITMAN was born in London in 1927. He spent part of his early life there, and subsequently lived in Dorset and Hertfordshire, returning to London to train in medicine at Westminster Hospital. After qualifying in 1949 he worked for a time in hospitals as a general physician, but after some years went to the Maudsley Hospital to become a psychiatrist. Later he joined a research team at Greylingwell Hospital, Chichester, where he remained until 1965. He then moved to Edinburgh where he is still working, currently as director of a research unit concerned with the distribution of psychological illness in the general population. Married, with two children. He began writing poetry as a young man, and has published in various periodicals.

WILLIAM LINDSAY was born in 1933 on a farm by Carrington, Midlothian, one of Scotland's prettiest villages. From his youth he was a member of the St. Andrew's Ambulance Association and in the army was Regimental Medical Sergeant of the 1st Battalion, Highland Light Infantry from 1952 to 1955. As such he was right hand man to several doctors and worked in hospitals in Malta and Tobruk. He is now a police chief inspector in London. Commenced writing late in 1974. His poems have appeared in a wide range of literary magazines. He was a diploma winner in both the 1977 and 1978 Scottish Open Poetry Cup Competition. His first collection, *Drawing on Experience,* was published by Outposts Publications in 1978.

EDWARD LOWBURY. Born in London 1913, the son of a general practitioner. At Oxford he held a medical scholarship, won two literary prizes (Newdigate and Matthew Arnold Memorial) and took degrees in physiology and medicine. After clinical studies at the London Hospital he served with the RAMC from 1943 to 1947. For 30 years Head of the Bacteriology Department of the MRC Burns Unit at Birmingham Accident Hospital. He is now Visiting Professor of Medical Microbiology in the University of Aston. He is a Doctor of Medicine (Oxford) and of Science (Aston, honorary); also Fellow of the Royal College of Physicians, Surgeons and Pathologists. As a writer, Edward Lowbury has produced a number of books of poems, most of them published by Chatto & Windus. His *Selected Poems* (Celtion) was published in 1978. He gave the third Keats Memorial Lecture in 1973 and in 1974 was elected a Fellow of the Royal Society of Literature.

RONALD MANN graduated from Westminster Hospital, London, in 1952 and spent five years in hospital practice, with emphasis on tuberculosis medicine, followed by a similar period in general practice before entering the pharmaceutical industry with which he has worked in medical research posts in Asia, the USA and Europe. Was given the London MD in 1969 for research on fibrinolysis on which he has written fairly extensively. Now lives in Sussex and is Medical Director of a pharmaceutical company in the UK. Has published in various magazines and his *Addingham Moorside* was published by Outposts Publications. His verse play, *Fiat Lux,* was performed by the Surrey Poetry Society.

E. MITTER was born in Burma and spent her earlier years there. Educated and pursued a medical career in Britain, with absences in France, Switzerland, Sweden and the USA. She is married to a Swiss Economist.

JENNY MORGAN was born in Newbridge, Gwent, in 1936. Since 1964 she has lived in Birmingham, where she now works as development officer for the National Association for the Welfare of Children in Hospital, an organisation which aims to increase awareness of the special emotional needs of children when they are in hospital and which is committed to the principle of parent participation in their care.

SIR RONALD ROSS was born in 1857 in India. Studied at St Bartholomew's Hospital. Won the Nobel Prize for Medicine in 1902 for his pioneer work on malaria, and the Royal Medal of the Royal Society in 1911.

HENRY SHORE. Qualified MD at Vienna University 1936. Worked for a year as House-Physician/Surgeon/Haematologist at the Allgemeines Krankenhaus, Vienna, unpaid but tolerated, because he was a Jew, and was then forbidden to follow his profession at all. Eked out an existence teaching music, English and Hebrew to private pupils. Came to England in 1938 but in 1940 was interned as an "enemy alien" and later shipped off to Australia for two years. When given the choice to return to Israel or England, chose the latter and was appointed House-Physician at the Emergency Hospital, Shotley Bridge. From 1945–1951 he had various posts as Medical Officer, Senior Houseman and Medical Registrar, and in 1951 he was appointed District Medical Officer in Uganda. Whilst there he discovered a new virus disease Onyong-nyong ("break-bone") fever. Wrote a thesis and collaborated with the East African Virus Research Institute. In 1961 he returned as Medical Officer of Health for Aldridge/Brownhills. Several collections of his poetry have been published by Outposts Publications. Dr Shore died in May, 1977, leaving a wife and two daughters.

VALERIE SINASON was born in 1946. She is married to a psychiatrist and has two children. She is currently a group worker with children having particular problems and stresses in an Inner London Junior School and concurrently studying the psychoanalytically orientated Child Observation Courses at the Tavistock Centre. She has written for *New Psychiatry, Health Team,* and *The Teacher* etc. and edits *Gallery,* a poetry magazine. Her own poems have appeared in *Outposts, Ambit, Little Word Machine, Palantir, Omens, Contemporary Women Poets* (Rondo) and other anthologies.

JUDITH SMALLSHAW was born in London 1935. A freelance journalist, as well as a poet, she writes for a medical newspaper. She has been married to a doctor for twenty years. Her two books, *Copper Farthings* and *By Fell, Tarn and Crag* were both published in 1978.

S. L. HENDERSON SMITH was born in North China 1919. Returned to China as a Medical Missionary in 1943, after Oxford and House jobs in Bath. Transferred to Central Africa (Belgian Congo) 1951, where he worked in a remote jungle hospital until 1954. In 1955 entered General Practice and has remained in this capacity since 1956 in Huddersfield. Has published seven volumes of poetry, most of them by Outposts Publications. An enthusiast for Voluntary Euthanasia, Conservation and Bee-keeping. Once said, "As a GP I have had to write poetry or go bonkers."

JILL THOMAS was born at Bristol in 1938. Educated at St Hilda's Convent, Whitby, and trained as a nurse at the Royal Informary, Edinburgh. After working as School Matron at a boys' prep school in Thanet for a year, she gave up work to raise a family. She subsequently served as Night Nurse for one year at Overley Hall, the local Sunshine Home for Blind Children, and since 1973 has been SRN District Sister with Salop Area Health Authority. She has contributed poems to a number of periodicals.

PATRICIA TORRINGTON was trained (SRN) at St Mary's General Hospital, Portsmouth from 1968–1971, going on to complete her postgraduate theatre experience there also. She left in 1972 to do industrial work, and then moved into the pharmaceutical world in 1973. She completed the ABPI examinations in 1974 and became involved in Medical Market Research. Her recent studies have included Hormones, Thrombolytic Treatments, New Trends in Arthritis, etc. She writes articles and short stories, as well as poetry.

GAEL TURNBULL was born in Edinburgh, 1928. Early education in the north of England and in Canada. Cambridge BA 1948. Qualified at the University of Pennsylvania in the United States, 1951. General practice for three years in Canada. Then hospital work in London and Worcester. Diploma in Anaesthetics 1957. Six years as consultant anaesthetist at the Ventura County General Hospital in Southern California. Returned to England in 1964 and since then has been in general practice in Worcester with hospital sessions in anaesthetics at Kidderminster General Hospital. Lives in Malvern. Married with three daughters. His principal publications: *A Trampoline: Poems of 1952–64* (Cape Goliard 1968), *Scantlings* (Cape Goliard 1976) and *If a Glance Could Be Enough* (Satis 1978). Was represented in *Children of Albion* and *British Poetry Since 1945.*

HENRY VAUGHAN (1622–95) was educated at Jesus College, Oxford, but left without a degree in order to study Law in London. He was an ardent Royalist

the Tavistock Centre. She has written for *New Psychiatry, Health Team,* and *The Teacher* etc. and edits *Gallery,* a poetry magazine. Her own poems have appeared in *Outposts, Ambit, Little Word Machine, Palantir, Omens, Contemporary Women Poets* (Rondo) and other anthologies.

JUDITH SMALLSHAW was born in London 1935. A freelance journalist, as well as a poet, she writes for a medical newspaper. She has been married to a doctor for twenty years. Her two books, *Copper Farthings* and *By Fell, Tarn and Crag* were both published in 1978.

S. L. HENDERSON SMITH was born in North China 1919. Returned to China as a Medical Missionary in 1943, after Oxford and House jobs in Bath. Transferred to Central Africa (Belgian Congo) 1951, where he worked in a remote jungle hospital until 1954. In 1955 entered General Practice and has remained in this capacity since 1956 in Huddersfield. Has published seven volumes of poetry, most of them by Outposts Publications. An enthusiast for Voluntary Euthanasia, Conservation and Bee-keeping. Once said, "As a GP I have had to write poetry or go bonkers."

JILL THOMAS was born at Bristol in 1938. Educated at St Hilda's Convent, Whitby, and trained as a nurse at the Royal Informary, Edinburgh. After working as School Matron at a boys' prep school in Thanet for a year, she gave up work to raise a family. She subsequently served as Night Nurse for one year at Overley Hall, the local Sunshine Home for Blind Children, and since 1973 has been SRN District Sister with Salop Area Health Authority. She has contributed poems to a number of periodicals.

PATRICIA TORRINGTON was trained (SRN) at St Mary's General Hospital, Portsmouth from 1968–1971, going on to complete her postgraduate theatre experience there also. She left in 1972 to do industrial work, and then moved into the pharmaceutical world in 1973. She completed the ABPI examinations in 1974 and became involved in Medical Market Research. Her recent studies have included Hormones, Thrombolytic Treatments, New Trends in Arthritis, etc. She writes articles and short stories, as well as poetry.

GAEL TURNBULL was born in Edinburgh, 1928. Early education in the north of England and in Canada. Cambridge BA 1948. Qualified at the University of Pennsylvania in the United States, 1951. General practice for three years in Canada. Then hospital work in London and Worcester. Diploma in Anaesthetics 1957. Six years as consultant anaesthetist at the Ventura County General Hospital in Southern California. Returned to England in 1964 and since then has been in general practice in Worcester with hospital sessions in anaesthetics at Kidderminster General Hospital. Lives in Malvern. Married with three daughters. His principal publications: *A Trampoline: Poems of 1952–64* (Cape Goliard 1968), *Scantlings* (Cape Goliard 1976) and *If a Glance Could Be Enough* (Satis 1978). Was represented in *Children of Albion* and *British Poetry Since 1945.*

HENRY VAUGHAN (1622–95) was educated at Jesus College, Oxford, but left without a degree in order to study Law in London. He was an ardent Royalist

them published by Chatto & Windus. His *Selected Poems* (Celtion) was published in 1978. He gave the third Keats Memorial Lecture in 1973 and in 1974 was elected a Fellow of the Royal Society of Literature.

RONALD MANN graduated from Westminster Hospital, London, in 1952 and spent five years in hospital practice, with emphasis on tuberculosis medicine, followed by a similar period in general practice before entering the pharmaceutical industry with which he has worked in medical research posts in Asia, the USA and Europe. Was given the London MD in 1969 for research on fibrinolysis on which he has written fairly extensively. Now lives in Sussex and is Medical Director of a pharmaceutical company in the UK. Has published in various magazines and his *Addingham Moorside* was published by Outposts Publications. His verse play, *Fiat Lux*, was performed by the Surrey Poetry Society.

E. MITTER was born in Burma and spent her earlier years there. Educated and pursued a medical career in Britain, with absences in France, Switzerland, Sweden and the USA. She is married to a Swiss Economist.

JENNY MORGAN was born in Newbridge, Gwent, in 1936. Since 1964 she has lived in Birmingham, where she now works as development officer for the National Association for the Welfare of Children in Hospital, an organisation which aims to increase awareness of the special emotional needs of children when they are in hospital and which is committed to the principle of parent participation in their care.

SIR RONALD ROSS was born in 1857 in India. Studied at St Bartholomew's Hospital. Won the Nobel Prize for Medicine in 1902 for his pioneer work on malaria, and the Royal Medal of the Royal Society in 1911.

HENRY SHORE. Qualified MD at Vienna University 1936. Worked for a year as House-Physician/Surgeon/Haematologist at the Allgemeines Krankenhaus, Vienna, unpaid but tolerated, because he was a Jew, and was then forbidden to follow his profession at all. Eked out an existence teaching music, English and Hebrew to private pupils. Came to England in 1938 but in 1940 was interned as an "enemy alien" and later shipped off to Australia for two years. When given the choice to return to Israel or England, chose the latter and was appointed House-Physician at the Emergency Hospital, Shotley Bridge. From 1945–1951 he had various posts as Medical Officer, Senior Houseman and Medical Registrar, and in 1951 he was appointed District Medical Officer in Uganda. Whilst there he discovered a new virus disease Onyong-nyong ("break-bone") fever. Wrote a thesis and collaborated with the East African Virus Research Institute. In 1961 he returned as Medical Officer of Health for Aldridge/Brownhills. Several collections of his poetry have been published by Outposts Publications. Dr Shore died in May, 1977, leaving a wife and two daughters.

VALERIE SINASON was born in 1946. She is married to a psychiatrist and has two children. She is currently a group worker with children having particular problems and stresses in an Inner London Junior School and concurrently studying the psychoanalytically orientated Child Observation Courses at and fought on the King's side in the Civil War. It is not entirely clear where he studied medicine, but he practised as a doctor at Brecknock and Newton by Usk. His two volumes of religious poetry, *Silex Scintillans,* were published in 1650 and 1655.

ANN WARD. Born 1928. State Registered Nurse, 1952, Blackburn. Married and brought up a daughter and two sons. She has worked as Staff Nurse for two years recently in Lancaster. Her poems have been published in a variety of magazines, etc, including *Outposts* and her first collection of poems was published by Outposts Publications in 1974.